APPETITE FOR PROFIT

dust record

APPETITE
FOR PROFIT

HOW
THE FOOD
INDUSTRY
UNDERMINES
OUR HEALTH
**AND HOW TO
FIGHT BACK**

MICHELE SIMON

NATION
BOOKS

APPETITE FOR PROFIT
How the Food Industry Undermines our Health and How to Fight Back

Published by
Nation Books
An Imprint of Avalon Publishing Group, Inc.
245 West 17th St., 11th Floor
New York, NY 10011
www.nationbooks.org

AVALON
publishing group incorporated

Nation Books is a co-publishing venture of the Nation Institute and Avalon Publishing Group Incorporated.

Library of Congress Cataloging-in-Publication Data

Cloth edition

ISBN-10: 1-56025-997-3
ISBN-13: 978-1-56025-997-8

Trade paperback edition

ISBN-10: 1-56025-932-9
ISBN-13: 978-1-56025-932-9

9 8 7 6 5 4 3 2 1

Book design by Maria E. Torres

Printed in the United States of America
Distributed by Publishers Group West

For my father,
who taught me
to take the road less traveled.

CONTENTS

Acknowledgments · ix

Introduction · xi

1 | Chapter 1: Anatomy of a Food Corporation:
Why We Can't Trust Them

21 | Chapter 2: Personal Responsibility, Energy Balance,
and Other Distractions

45 | Chapter 3: Freedom from Choice:
Distortions of All-American Values

67 | Chapter 4: Nutriwashing Fast Food

91 | Chapter 5: Nutriwashing Processed Foods

117 | Chapter 6: "Responsible Marketing" to Kids

143 | Chapter 7: Exposing Government Complicity

167 | Chapter 8: Co-opting the Science

195 | Chapter 9: Eating in the Dark: Nutrition Labeling in
Restaurants

219 | Chapter 10: Battling Big Food in Schools

245 | Chapter 11: Regulating Junk Food Marketing to
Children

273 | Chapter 12: Scapegoating Lawyers

299 | Chapter 13: The Bigger Picture

Appendix 1: Anti-Glossary · 323

Appendix 2: Guide to Industry Groups and Spin Doctoring · 331

Appendix 3: Myth vs. Reality: Nutrition Labeling at Fast-Food
and Other Chain Restaurants · 339

Appendix 4: Taking Back Our Schools • 343

Appendix 5: Protect Your Legal Rights • 349

Appendix 6: Resources for Positive Change • 353

Endnotes • 361

Index • 381

ACKNOWLEDGMENTS

I am extremely fortunate to benefit from the generosity of many wonderful friends, dedicated colleagues, and supportive family members. The first person to encourage me to write this book was Anna Lappé, to whom I am forever grateful. Patti Breitman patiently and expertly guided me through the entire publishing process and landed me with my wonderful agent Matthew Carnicelli. Matthew saw the importance of this project and stalwartly refused to give up until we found the right home in Nation Books. My editor Carl Bromley was always a delight, making this first-time author feel completely at ease.

Numerous colleagues too many to list have offered me guidance and inspiration. I am especially grateful to Marion Nestle, Ellen Fried, Susan Linn, Alan Kanner, Richard Daynard, Jason Smith, David Yosifon, Susan Roberts, Gary Ruskin, and Linda Bacon for their encouragement and expert feedback.

I was blessed with the generosity of several research volunteers who dutifully tracked down corporate shenanigans, including Christine Treveloni, Maida Genser, Mark Mayada, and especially Layla Azimi.

One of the nice fringe benefits of teaching at a law school

is tapping into some the best and brightest young minds. I am grateful to University of California, Hastings College of the Law students Lisa Sofio, Rachelle Acuna-Narvaez, Shane Glynn, and Amy Leung for their excellent legal research assistance.

In the special mention category, two names stand out. Colleen Patrick-Goudreau is a dear friend who helped me stay focused under tremendous time pressure. Richard Ganis went far beyond the call of friendship duty both in lending his expert editing skills and in spending hours talking through many of the book's theoretical underpinnings.

Throughout my life my mother Florence Peloquin has served as a role model who instilled in me the core values reflected in this book: integrity and fairness. My stepmother Celeste Simon is also a source of unwavering support.

No author could ask for a more supportive life partner than Ross Turner. He cheered me on lovingly, listened patiently, and made dinner willingly. I am also grateful to my wonderful stepdaughter Lynden Turner for understanding why I was constantly working, and for liking tofu and broccoli.

Finally, I want to thank the many dedicated grassroots advocates and local politicians who generously gave of their precious time in sharing their experiences fighting against Big Food, and for constantly keeping me updated on both their victories and defeats.

This book is my attempt to give them something back.

INTRODUCTION

Digging Our Graves with Knives and Forks

Most Americans take for granted the mind-boggling amount of unhealthy food currently available anywhere, anytime, from entire grocery store aisles devoted to chips, soda, and ice cream to the endless fast-food chains found on every block and at every highway exit. Nowadays you can't even walk into a bookstore without being tempted by mocha lattes and megamuffins. But this ubiquitous availability of food is really a very recent development in human history.

For the first hundreds of thousands of years of human evolution, our ancestors struggled to scrape together enough food just to survive. Because in nature foods high in salt, sugar, and fat were also high in nutrients and calories, we evolved to seek out these flavors. Since food was so scarce, we also evolved to store excess calories as fat. Humans are hardwired to prepare for famine. Humans who survived the hard times—by storing fat efficiently—were rewarded with longevity and passed their "thrifty genes" on to their children.[1]

Now, thanks to industrialization, transportation, and the commercialization of the food supply, we live in a world where fatty, sugary, and salty foods—stripped of nutrients during factory processing—are in abundance. The ubiquitous animal products Americans eat in no way resemble the lean meats our ancestors occasionally found in nature. Today's industrialized meat, eggs, and dairy products are artificially high in fat, hormones, and other additives. Average annual consumption of cheese alone increased 287 percent between the 1950s and 2000, mostly in processed and prepared food.[2] Also, clever manufacturers have made processed food artificially stimulating by isolating particular chemicals that cause pleasure reactions, creating new "foods" that don't exist in nature and ensuring that we stay hooked.

For most Americans, these nutrient-deficient factory-made pseudofoods have replaced the real food that Mother Nature intended us to eat: mostly plant-based unprocessed foods such as whole grains, legumes, and fresh produce that are packed with the fiber and nutrients our bodies need. A closer look at how Americans eat gives us some idea of the problem: 51 percent of our calories come from processed foods, 42 percent from meat, eggs, or dairy, and a paltry 7 percent from vegetables, fruits, legumes, whole grains, nuts, and seeds— foods that prevent disease and are optimum for overall health.[3] By comparison, early humans obtained 65 percent of their food energy from a wide variety of fruits and vegetables.[4] Government surveys consistently confirm that Americans aren't eating anywhere near the government's daily recommended five to nine servings of fruits and vegetables.[5] And our favorite "vegetable"? French fries.[6]

Another huge change is our obsession with sugary beverages. Sounds crazy, but humans used to just drink water. The nation's steep increase of sugar consumption directly follows the rise in soft drinks. Soft drinks are the biggest source of calories and provide more than one-third of all refined sugars in the American diet. Over the past sixty years, soft drink production has increased tenfold; consumption has doubled since 1971. Soda provides the average teenage boy with about fifteen teaspoons of refined sugar per day and girls about ten teaspoons.[7]

Also, most of the added salt, sugar, and fat Americans consume is hidden, either in processed foods or by restaurants when we eat out. For example, about 90 percent of salt intake comes from food processing, preparation, and flavoring. Only 10 percent is intrinsic to the food itself. Interestingly, the few remaining hunter-gatherer cultures that don't have access to commercial salt show no signs of high blood pressure.[8]

All this ready access to highly processed food is taking its toll. Government figures show that our daily caloric intake increased by a staggering 24.5 percent, or 530 calories, between 1970 and 2000.[9] Uncle Sam estimates we eat 2,700 calories a day; the recommended average is 2,000.[10] By overeating (and drinking), humans are constantly storing excess calories, which is not at all what nature intended. And all this has happened in a blink of an eye in the course of human history. It's no wonder we're suffering the effects; the human body cannot possibly adapt so rapidly. We've turned our evolutionary protection on its head, and a steady diet of Big Macs, Doritos, Chips Ahoy, and Coke is making Americans sick.

For years, nutrition advocates were the only ones talking about this problem. But in December 2001, the media, policy makers, and the general public got a huge wake-up call with the release of the U.S. surgeon general's "call to action" on obesity. It was this report that gave us the now familiar statistic that close to two-thirds of Americans are overweight or obese.[11] Today's generation of children may be the first to have shorter lives than their parents. According to one prediction, nearly half the children in North and South America will be overweight by 2010.[12] Especially troubling are the rising obesity trends in developing countries as Western foods are increasingly marketed overseas. In an ironic twist of global "progress," the number of overweight people around the world—1.1 billion—now roughly equals those who are underweight, with both populations suffering from malnutrition and disease.[13] But more important than obesity are the increased health risks associated with poor diet, which include heart disease, type 2 diabetes, hypertension, stroke, and certain cancers. Even thin people aren't immune to the negative impacts of eating too much of the wrong foods. Cardiovascular disease is by far the nation's number-one killer, claiming more than 900,000 lives in 2002.[14] The total cost associated with such health problems was estimated at $117 billion in 2000.[15]

Setting the PR Wheels in Motion

Since the surgeon general's report, obesity has become the most visible marker of America's diet-related health problems, resulting in a public and political firestorm. At the center of the controversy is the simple question: who is to blame? With food marketers spending upwards of $36 billion a year to peddle its habit-forming products,[16] it's no wonder experts and policy makers alike are starting to ask tough questions. Adding to the industry's PR nightmare, children have become a focal point in the debate. With rising rates of childhood obesity and diabetes (we can no longer call Type 2 diabetes "adult onset diabetes"), more and more people are asking why companies like McDonald's and Coca-Cola are targeting such a vulnerable population.

Not willing to take all the finger-pointing lying down, the major food companies are currently engaged in a massive public relations campaign designed to protect their images and, ultimately, their bottom lines. Corporations concerned with their brand images are tripping over each other trying to spin themselves as "part of the solution" when it comes to solving this public health crisis. As we will see, their PR methods vary and include seemingly altruistic acts such as donations for exercise programs, selling allegedly healthier products, and "improved" marketing policies toward children.

But in the end, their promises simply amount to a lot of hot air. The PR campaign is designed to maintain profits by accomplishing two important goals: shoring up positive public images and deflecting the threat of government regulation and lawsuits. Adding insult to injury, while food companies are performing cartwheels to make you believe they are "doing the right thing," behind the scenes, corporate lobbyists are conducting business as usual. As a result of these efforts, virtually every commonsense health policy, such as getting soda out of schools, has been either blocked, delayed, or significantly compromised. Understanding how the major players operate can go a long way toward fighting back.

Countering Industry Rhetoric and Lobbying Tactics

At the heart of any public discourse is how the issues are

"framed." Political frames are words or ideas that bring to mind broader concepts in ways that are often symbolic. Cognitive research shows that to make sense of the world we use stored knowledge in the form of pictures in our heads. The food industry understands the power of shaping the public debate and hires highly trained PR experts to coordinate media strategy and develop key talking points. But most health advocates are still stuck in defensive mode, allowing the media and food companies to frame the debate. It's critical that we be ready with the best responses to corporate arguments, as well as go on the offensive in describing the issues. While framing is important, underneath the rhetoric is a massive imbalance in power and democratic process that cannot be overcome with words alone.

Learning how to pierce through industry rhetoric can be a powerful tool to expose corporate spin. A food lobbyist's main goal is to provide any distraction, misdirection, or obfuscation possible to avoid talking about corporate accountability. The goal of all industry rhetoric, activities, and lobbying is to keep government out of their business while maintaining the media focus on individual behavior change as the true solution to America's health problems. While modifying individual eating behavior is important, the tools in this book will help advocates focus the debate on policy solutions that hold industry accountable for their role in perpetuating the public health crisis.

Policies aimed at changing food-industry marketing practices are critical because "personal responsibility" doesn't occur in a vacuum. Our food choices are heavily influenced by a complex set of laws that often have more to do with political power than with public health. For example, the federal government provides corn growers with massive subsidies, which results in the production of high fructose corn syrup, the cheap sweetener found in almost every processed food and a significant contributor to our health problems. Thanks in part to corporate lobbying, our federal food policies have yet to catch up with nutrition science.

Moreover, educational campaigns such as the government's "5 a Day" program (which encourages people to eat five to nine servings of fruits and vegetables per day) are woefully ineffective in bringing about behavioral change. How can we tell people to eat more vegetables if the only place to buy food in their neighborhood is the corner liquor store, as is the case for many Americans? How can we teach children about good nutrition while we continue to peddle soda, chips, and candy in schools? Such problems are best solved through effective policy change. Most public health experts now recognize the critical role of government and society at large in shaping our food choices. This is precisely why food companies are lobbying against any legislative efforts to improve the "food environment." Food companies know that as long as they keep the nation focused on "education" and "individual choice," the status quo is virtually guaranteed. But actually changing the way that food is produced, sold, and marketed represents a genuine threat to the corporate bottom line.

Because of this threat, food companies are desperate to maintain control over policymaking. Corporations know they cannot win policy battles by engaging in a genuine debate on the substance of the issues, so they often resort to the kind of underhanded political tactics used by Big Tobacco. These strategies include: forming scientific "front groups" (groups that do the dirty work that image-conscious companies shy away from, and that generally don't reveal their funding sources or are otherwise deceptive about their motives), buying off health experts, making incongruous arguments, and the old standby: backroom political dealing. When all else fails, corporate shills resort to shooting the messenger. My colleagues and I are often marginalized as "the food police," out-of-control zealots with a "hidden agenda" to get "Big Brother" to take away your God-given right to Big Macs and Big Gulps. The goal of these attacks is to once again detract attention from the heart of the matter: that corporations control most of our food choices. Once you realize that most industry arguments are disingenuous, hypocritical, misleading, or downright false, it's quite easy to expose them as self-serving statements designed to obfuscate the real issues.

Something's Amiss

I am not sure if every writer has a eureka moment when she just knows the book she has to write. For me, it came in June 2004 while I was attending the *Time*/ABC News Summit on Obesity in Williamsburg, Virginia. The two media giants gathered several hundred experts to forge "solutions" to America's expanding waistline. Then U.S. secretary of health and human services Tommy Thompson delivered the keynote address in his customary cheerleading style. He praised all the major food companies for being "responsible" corporate citizens, singling out Coca-Cola for improving its school-based marketing policy.

Then, during the question-and-answer session, an amazing thing happened. A state representative from Indiana named Charlie Brown stood up to ask: if Coca-Cola was such a responsible citizen, then why had the company sent five lobbyists to Brown's state capitol to kill his school nutrition bill, a measure that would have required only 50 percent of school beverages to be healthy? Suddenly, Thompson's jocular manner turned defensive as he stammered his reply: "Well, I don't know anything about that, but if it happens again, you call me."

Right.

At that moment I became aware of a troubling dichotomy: on the one hand, the nation's top health official was telling us that Corporate America was taking care of the problem. But on the ground in state legislatures, reality wasn't reflecting the rhetoric. Upon further investigation, I confirmed my suspicions that Representative Brown wasn't the only well-meaning local politician finding himself at the receiving end of industry lobbying against commonsense nutrition policies. But the extent of the corporate duplicity and hypocrisy was even worse than I had imagined.

Who's Who in Big Food

For the purposes of this book, it helps to divide food-industry players into two main sectors: restaurant and packaged-food. My selection process (whom I deem "Big Food") within those two groups was fairly simple. I chose to focus on companies recognized as leaders of their respective categories, companies whose brand names are familiar to every household in America. And they are, not coincidentally, the companies that have been the most vocal in positioning themselves as "part of the solution" when it comes to obesity. These corporations include: Coca-Cola, PepsiCo, Kraft Foods, General Mills, and McDonald's.

In addition to individual companies, I have also chosen to highlight several trade associations and front groups engaged in various lobbying activities on behalf of Big Food. By pooling large sums of money to support these third-party organizations, individual corporations gain greater lobbying power. Some organizations are easy to spot, such as trade associations, while others give the impression they are "grass-roots" or hide behind scientific-sounding names. Here are a few examples of those we will meet.

Grocery Manufacturers Association

The GMA's 140 members consist of every major food manufacturer, accounting for combined annual sales of more than $680 billion.[17] GMA is on record as opposing virtually every state bill that would restrict the sale of junk food or soda in schools, in addition to other nutrition policies.

National Restaurant Association

The powerful National Restaurant Association's sixty thousand member companies represent more than 300,000 dining establishments.[18] The NRA strongly opposes providing nutrition information, and is determined to block access to the courtroom by consumers who might be harmed by eating its members' food.

Center for Consumer Freedom

Despite its populist name, this organization does not represent consumers at all. Rather, it's a lobbying front for the restaurant, food, beverage, and alcohol industries. Employing attack dog–style tactics, CCF consistently portrays nutrition-policy advocates as "food cops" and radicals.

The American Council for Fitness and Nutrition

Despite its official, objective-sounding name, ACFN is actually backed by Big Food's heaviest hitters, including Coca-Cola and Kraft Foods, along with several trade associations such as the Association of National Advertisers, GMA, and NRA. In addition to outright lobbying and cheerleading for its member companies, ACFN publishes industry-friendly articles in both the academic press and the general media, usually without revealing its corporate backing.

David vs. Goliath

In later chapters, we will meet numerous public health heroes fighting against powerful food-industry lobbying. They include people like Representative Brown of Indiana, who stood up to Secretary Thompson by not letting him get away with describing Coca-Cola as a "responsible citizen." Certain states, such as California, Connecticut, Maine, and New York, have been national leaders in forging nutrition policy, stepping in to fill the void of activity in Washington.

I wish I could describe nutrition-advocacy efforts as well funded, well coordinated, and well organized, but that's just not the case. On the national level, there are precious few groups even raising the alarm about the problems of diet-related illness. And those who do tend to focus on the safer "educational" approaches as opposed to hard-hitting policy. Compared to other social issues, such as the environment, only a few national advocacy organizations work on nutrition. Such groups include the Center for Science in the Public Interest, the Physicians Committee for Responsible Medicine, and Commercial Alert.

Making up for the lack of sufficient national resources is a vocal grassroots movement. Those who seek, for example, to improve school food believe that schools should be a safe haven from corporate messages to get kids to eat the wrong foods. Across the nation, parents, teachers, health professionals, and others are taking action.

I am constantly encouraged by those dedicated to making healthy eating the norm for everyone. I wrote this book to help this growing grassroots movement, and in the hope of inspiring others to join the effort. Armed with the right tools, we can begin to fight back. Ultimately, finding the best solutions requires first correctly identifying the underlying causes of the problem.

1

Anatomy of
a Food Corporation:
Why We Can't Trust Them

B ig Food is facing a public relations nightmare. The United
States is in the midst of a growing epidemic of diet-related
health problems, including obesity, heart disease, and diabetes. Experts have written extensively about our "toxic food
environment," caused in large part by overzealous corporate
marketing strategies.[1] With the nation now firmly entrenched
in a public health crisis, researchers, policy makers, and the
media are looking for answers.

Food makers are reacting in various ways, but the motivation
behind their responses is always the same: to spin a positive corporate image and stave off threats of government regulation and
private litigation over their products and practices.

Too many people—including nutrition advocates and
lawmakers—think that solving the nation's diet-related
health problems is simply a matter of persuading food manufacturers to change their behavior. They mistakenly believe

that somewhere deep within their souls, corporations have a "conscience" and can "do the right thing" (e.g., provide "healthier" products or stop marketing to children), even if that means a loss of profit. But in fact, we really cannot expect food companies to be the guardians of public health.

Corporations 101

Sometimes I'm charged with having an "anticorporate agenda," or people misinterpret my views as suggesting that food companies are engaged in some sort of evil conspiracy. Neither allegation is true. I have nothing against profit-making per se, except when it does harm. I have simply come to realize that under our current economic system it's not a corporation's job to protect the public health.

No particular political mind-set is needed to recognize that corporations are in business to make money. The positions that I take in describing how food companies operate are guided by understanding basic corporate imperatives. Once you appreciate that corporations must abide by certain rules to remain competitive, it becomes much easier to recognize and predict their behavior. Here, then, is a guide to understanding how corporations think.

The scruples of a doorknob

The biggest mistake most people make about corporations is seeing them as just people making decisions. Unlike most people—who have consciences and act (we hope) on the basis of some set of moral principles—a corporation is a fundamentally amoral institution. Of course, corporations are made up of people, but the decisions of individual corporate actors are not guided by precepts of right and wrong, but rather by a set of fiduciary principles that have little to do with personal morality and everything to do with growing profits. Colleagues have asked me, in relation to some of the more appalling marketing strategies, questions like: "How do corporate executives sleep at night?" To which I reply: "They sleep just fine; their jobs depend on it." In fact, managers who willfully allow the bottom line to suffer to protect the public good can be sued by company shareholders for breach of their legal obligations.

To make matters worse, the Supreme Court has granted corporations certain "personhood" rights, such as limited free speech, which allows companies to advertise largely unhampered by government regulations. However, despite operating under the legal fiction of personhood, corporations do not bear the same responsibilities as people. In his excellent book and accompanying documentary film *The Corporation*, author Joel Bakan likens corporations to psychopaths, noting their freedom from the obligation to abide by the same moral and ethical constraints as everybody else. This point is underscored by legal analysts Frank H. Easterbrook and Daniel R. Fishel, who note: "Only people have moral obligations. Corporations can no more be said to have moral obligations than does a building, an organizational chart, or a contract."[2] In other words, a corporation's ability to "do the right thing" is circumscribed by its very organizing principles, which command it to act exclusively in its own self-interest. Because corporations have no moral obligations to society, we cannot expect food companies to "do the right thing"; nor should we believe them when they claim that they are. It's simply not in the nature of the corporate form.

Show me the money

The most important guiding principle of every corporation is maximizing profits for shareholders. Because doing so is legally required of corporate executives, profit must be the ultimate measure of all business decisions. This imperative is brought home by none other than Nobel Prize–winning economist and free market champion Milton Friedman, who asserts that "the only social responsibility of business is to make a profit."[3] While corporate managers shouldn't completely ignore social concerns, Friedman says, managers are to act on them only when it would result in increased profits. The truth is that under a free enterprise system, corporations cannot place moral or ethical concerns ahead of profit maximization because doing so risks being driven out of business by competing firms that are not similarly plagued by social conscience. Therefore, despite corporate attempts to proclaim their desire to act responsibly, the underlying drive for profit maximization always remains.

The food industry is just another example of this model. It is vitally important to understand the economic constraints under which a food company operates. Many people mistakenly believe that companies can simply stop marketing certain products out of the goodness of their hearts. The truth is that every decision a company makes that might undercut profits in one part of the business must be made up for somewhere else.

Grow or die

Driven by this basic profit-above-all-else directive, corporations are mandated, in effect, to "grow or die," a rule also called "the growth imperative."

Of course, a food maker is no different from any other corporation operating in a free market economy. However, food companies face special challenges when it comes to obeying the market's growth imperative: because there's a limit—in theory, anyway—to the number of calories humans can consume, competition is especially fierce among food makers for the finite pool of money that consumers can spend.

Lee Allen is a financial analyst who has been closely following the obesity epidemic and is concerned that food companies are not taking the threat seriously enough. He explained to me that the growth principle is especially important because food companies can't grow any faster than population growth. "Food has very little internal growth, and so food companies are always fighting for market share. That always leads to aggressive marketing."[4]

Accordingly, food sellers have developed a staggering array of marketing gimmicks and promotions to entice consumers to push their biological food-consumption limits. In an effort to make products like Chips Ahoy Candy Blasts cookies and Frosted Chocolate Fudge Pop-Tarts staples of every American household, food companies spend as much as $36 billion a year on marketing. Allen says that consolidation among food companies in recent decades has made competition even fiercer, with much more at stake for fewer and larger companies. "As long as large, wealthy companies are competing on a grand scale, they are going to try to get people to buy more of their product, which isn't particularly a good solution to the obesity problem. Companies are going to continue to load it up with salt, sugar, and fat."[5]

Exploiting nature and public health

When you get right down to it, purveyors of food and other commodities are in the business of transforming the natural world and bringing it to market in the form of manufactured goods. Trees are turned into paper, houses, furniture; crude oil is converted into saleable energy, plastics, agrochemicals, and so on. As author Jerry Mander notes, this drive to incessantly exploit nature recognizes no limits and is thus inherently eco-destructive: "Extracting resources from nature everywhere on Earth and reprocessing them at an ever-quickening pace is intrinsic to corporate existence. The net effect is the corporate ravaging of nature."[6] Guided by this directive, food companies refashion natural nourishment into industrial products bearing little resemblance to anything humans were designed to eat, and persuade people to consume as much as possible—public health consequences be damned.

Food companies like Kraft, McDonald's, and Coca-Cola maximize profit by taking raw materials such as wheat, potatoes, salt, and sugar, pulverizing them and combining them with a chemical soup of additives; at the other end of the factory, out comes a wide array of "consumer products." So why can't companies just make money selling "healthier prod-ucts"? Because companies make more money selling unhealthy food. Truly healthy food doesn't come in a box. As I will discuss, we cannot expect food companies to "make healthier products." It simply cannot be done, and it certainly cannot be done in a way that both maximizes profits and ben-efits public health.

Someone else will pay

An important way in which corporations maintain high profits is by "externalizing costs." This means that others (communities, government agencies, individuals, whoever) must bear the burden of, and responsibility for, the harm that profit-making activities inflict on society. One accounting expert estimates that in 1995 alone U.S. corporations would have had to shell out $3.5 trillion if required to pay for all of the externalized costs (e.g., health-care expenses incurred as a result of work-related injuries, unsafe products, and pollu-tion) that their business activities generated—a figure four times greater than the $822 billion they earned in profits that year.[7] Too often, people mistakenly think that if food compa-nies just saw the impact that the obesity epidemic is having on health-care costs, for example, they would change their busi-ness practices. But food makers need not be concerned about the negative public health consequences associated with the over consumption of their products. In their minds, those are someone else's problems.

Corporations don't commit suicide

For all these reasons, we should be very suspicious when a

company talks about scaling back the production or marketing of certain foods in the name of public health. A corporation that stops (or reduces) manufacturing a profitable product or targeting a lucrative market risks going out of business. As financial analyst Lee Allen explains:

> Companies generally don't commit suicide. They generally don't cut off marketing plans to targeted markets. They don't shrink product lines; they don't remove products for the public good. They can't. The shareholders don't want it; they are not advocating cutting back anything.[8]

So rather than make significant changes and risk falling prey to the competition, food makers initiate only marginal, largely cosmetic changes to their traditional business practices—and then greatly exaggerate the benefits of these efforts for maximum PR effect.

Fear factor: countering negative PR

Indeed, with all the criticism getting directed their way, food manufacturers are becoming more and more concerned about maintaining positive public images. Allen explains that food companies are extremely sensitive to any criticism of their motivations because they rely on the trust and goodwill of the American people: "Companies like McDonald's, Coke, and Pepsi want to keep an image of being pro-kids, pro-family, and pro-America."[9] They've also been anxious to portray their products as not at all harmful, and to pitch some of them, at least, as healthful. As Allen details:

Companies are scared of people being discouraged from consuming their products. They are making lots of money selling products that critics are increasingly saying aren't healthy. It's worse than if you're making a fishing lure that doesn't catch fish, it's like making a plane that falls out of the sky. You're supposed to eat this stuff, right?[10]

In the end, of course, all the hype about healthy products and corporate responsibility has one basic aim: counteracting bad press that could result in loss of revenue and markets.

When Doing Right Is Really Wrong

At this point, you may be saying to yourself, so what if food corporations are only making minimal, superficial changes in the interest of safeguarding their bottom lines. At least they're doing something, right? Isn't it a good thing that companies are improving their products, even if only marginally? Isn't this a step in the right direction? Not necessarily. Plenty of food makers have opted not to position themselves as "part of the solution" to the current diet-related public health crisis. Major companies such as Burger King and Kellogg (both of whom heavily market junk food to children) have pretty much thumbed their noses at their critics, preferring to conduct business as usual instead. Because the marketing efforts of these food-industry players are rather conventional (and have been amply explored elsewhere), I've chosen not to focus on them.

Rather, my decision to write this book was motivated in large part by my concern that certain leading food companies, such as Kraft, McDonald's, and General Mills, have launched massive PR campaigns aimed at convincing policy makers— and indeed all Americans—that they are committed to making substantive changes that will redound to the benefit of the nation's health. The reality, though, is far different. As I will show, these moves promise to make things worse, not better, for consumers and society.

Why We Don't Let Foxes Guard Henhouses

A major goal of the PR maneuvering that we'll examine in the following chapters is aimed at persuading legislators and concerned citizens that government oversight of the food industry is unnecessary and that "self-regulation" is the answer to all problems. In making their case for this approach, food makers insist that they can be trusted to police themselves and behave as "responsible corporate citizens"—even when it comes to controversial issues such as junk food marketing to children. The idea is to keep government regulators at bay at all costs.

There are several problems with the self-regulation model of "reform," but they all boil down to this: corporations cannot be trusted. Since they are only in it for the money, short of bribery or outright coercion, how can they possibly be expected to do the right thing? As Joel Bakan eloquently elaborates in *The Corporation*, self-regulation:

> rests on the suspect premise that corporations will respect social and environmental interests without being compelled by government to do so. No one would seriously suggest that individuals should regulate

themselves, that laws against murder, assault, and theft are unnecessary because people are socially responsible. Yet oddly, we are asked to believe that corporate persons—institutional psychopaths who lack any sense of moral conviction and who have the power and motivation to cause harm and devastation in the world—should be left free to govern themselves.[11]

Eye on quarterly earnings

Because self-regulation by definition means that corporate behavior is voluntary, the company can decide to shift gears at any time based on external economic pressures. For example, in March 2004, the restaurant chain Ruby Tuesday decided to place nutrition information on its menus. The move earned founder and CEO Sandy Beall much positive publicity, including a "hero" award at that year's *Time*/ABC News Summit on Obesity. And yet just a few months later, the company retracted the policy for reasons that are still unclear. Perhaps including nutrition data on its menus was proving too costly for Ruby Tuesday's accountants. Or maybe sales of its Cheddar Bison Burgers, MegaNachos, and Crispy Buffalo Wontons dipped as a result of the new menu data. Either way, access to more information may be good for public health, but it can also be bad for business. Once a voluntary change negatively impacts a corporation's bottom line, the policy soon becomes a fleeting moment in history. That's why laws are needed to require companies to change their irresponsible business practices.

The fox's less-than-objective viewpoint

When a company gets to police itself, it has an inherent

conflict of interest in the outcome. A corporation cannot possibly be objective in determining optimum health standards. In a world of industry self-regulation, self-appointed corporate guardians decide what's best. This "hands-off" approach lacks any semblance of democratic decision-making (which still exists, in theory anyway, in the political realm). Where is the opportunity for public participation and deliberation? Food companies claim to welcome such scrutiny and insist that their expert advisory boards set "objective" standards for their policies. But as we will see, these so-called experts are in fact bought and paid for, and their conclusions certainly are not subject to anything like public debate and discussion.

Who's minding the store?

Who, then, are food makers accountable to when they initiate their privately administered public health policies? Who is overseeing their promises and making sure they follow through on them? Given that the deregulatory political climate of the early 1980s has become a way of life in Washington, certainly not the federal government. Over the past three decades, Uncle Sam has gradually and conspicuously exempted itself from its responsibility to hold corporations responsible for their actions.

Consider, for example, McDonald's 2002 promise to remove artery-clogging trans fat from its cooking oil. This decision earned the company many glowing accolades and an enormous PR boost. Yet as of this writing, fours years later, McDonald's has failed to fulfill its pledge and has suffered no penalties for this inaction from federal regulators. Self-regulation perpetuates such lack of accountability.

Only adding to the confusion

Another problem with self-regulation is the potential for increased confusion in the marketplace due to lack of standardization. Food companies are now free to craft their own nutrition guidelines, leaving consumers without any clear guidance from federal regulators on how to assess these claims. So now consumers—many of whom are already extremely bewildered by nutrition—are expected to figure it out for themselves. For example, we are seeing various new corporate "seal of approval" nutrition programs, which are impossible to evaluate without the benefit of any government-issued, universally recognized criteria.

Case Study in Corporate Irresponsibility: Big Soda's Shameless Publicity Stunt

The food industry provides us with numerous examples of how self-regulation has failed. Let's take a closer look at one clever corporate PR campaign disguised as policy to drive home the point. In August 2005, the American Beverage Association (ABA)—apparently feeling the heat from state legislatures, litigation threats, and a rising tide of grass-roots school-nutrition advocacy—decided that it was time to show the world that it really does care. With much fanfare, the ABA announced a new school-based policy "aimed at providing lower calorie and/or nutritious beverages to schools and limiting the availability of soft drinks."[12] To maximize the PR punch, the declaration was made at the annual meeting of the National Conference of State Legislatures. The ABA had been lobbying against state bills to improve school nutrition for years, so its selection of this audience for its initial pitch was no accident: the group was well aware of exactly whom it was wooing.

As a PR maneuver, the proclamation paid off well, precipitating an immediate rash of newspaper accounts with headlines such as "Soft Drink Industry Takes High Road,"[13] "Schools Get Ally in Soda Issue: Drink Makers,"[14] and "U.S. Beverage Industry Praised for Helping in Childhood Obesity Battle."[15] Many months later the decree continued to circulate in the press, where it was referred to as a fait accompli, even though it remained little more than words on paper.

A policy with lots of (PR) chops but no teeth

In fact, the ABA's school-based beverage policy never actually took hold. This makes sense when you realize that the ABA is just a trade association. As such, it does not directly oversee the sale of soft drinks in schools. Rather, beverages are sold to schools through local distributors, which operate under the jurisdiction of their individual parent companies. These controlling firms have the ultimate say regarding which products are made available to schools and under what terms. Moreover, the ABA proclamation is only voluntary and has no government enforcement or oversight mechanism. The ABA conceded that "the success of the policy is dependent on voluntary implementation of it by individual beverage companies and by school officials."[16]

The ABA school decree is anemic in other ways, too. For example, it applies only to vending machines, and imposes no restrictions on other venues where drinks are marketed in schools (e.g., in school canteens and at sporting events). Also, the policy applies only to new school contracts; it can be amended to old agreements only with the consent of both parties. But why would a soda company agree to change an existing contract voluntarily if doing so could hurt it financially?

An end run around legislative action

Let's be honest. The real aim of the ABA's pronouncement was to beat state legislators to the punch and initiate a beverage policy with the convenient advantage of being exceedingly friendly to industry interests. The move also enabled soda makers to position themselves as being "responsive" to lawmakers' efforts to pass school-based soda legislation—bills that create an enormous PR headache for industry when exposed in the popular press. This point was even acknowledged by a leading food-industry publication, *Vending Market Watch*, which noted: "This new policy is clearly designed to counteract criticism from consumer activists and politicians who say the beverage industry is profiting at children's expense."[17]

Other media outlets characterized the policy as representing a complete about-face from the ABA's earlier strenuous opposition to the idea of imposing any restrictions on in-school soda purchases. For example, an editorial in the *Atlanta Journal-Constitution* (Coca-Cola's hometown paper) opined: "The announcement this week by the American Beverage Association represents a reversal by the industry, which had been fighting legislative efforts to ban soft drinks from school vending machines."[18] For its part, the ABA insisted that its policy was not intended to replace any existing regulations (which it couldn't, legally, anyway).

Curiously, however, it gave no indication that its members would stop lobbying against school-nutrition legislation. So where's the reversal in policy?

In the months following the ABA's announcement, there were plenty of signs that its plan to stave off state legislation on in-school soda was working like a charm. Iowa lawmakers, for example, rejected a bill aimed at removing soda from schools. Tom Vilsack, the state's Democratic governor, supported the move and applauded the ABA for its leadership in "taking pop out of machines located in elementary and middle schools."[19] In Massachusetts, legislators introduced a measure that basically mirrored the ABA's voluntary policy.[20] But why would we need a bill to legislate what the ABA has said they are already doing voluntarily?

A multimillion-dollar PR campaign

To ensure the success of its crafty publicity stunt, the ABA announced a multimillion-dollar campaign "to run print and broadcast advertising to educate the public about the new policy."[21] Of course, spending this kind of cash had less to do with educating the public than with securing positive PR spin. If the policy was truly reflective of a desire to be "part of the solution" to childhood obesity, why would the ABA need to advertise it? Wouldn't just making improvements in schools be reward enough? What possible purpose could an ad campaign serve, other than to promote soda companies as responsible and caring corporate citizens? If this tactic sounds eerily familiar, it should. Taking a page right out of Big Tobacco's playbook, Big Soda spent more money on promoting themselves as responsible than on actually being responsible.

A press release does not equal policy

The ABA would clearly not have invested so generously in its school proposal if it did not expect handsome rewards. The announcement garnered enormous traction, not only in the press but also among policy makers. Even some of my colleagues were impressed. One noted that while nothing has actually *changed* as a result of the new policy, the ABA's efforts to create the *perception* that beverage sellers are committed to doing something meaningful to address the problem of in-school soda sales was enormously successful at the PR level.

In May 2006, apparently recognizing that the 2005 press release hadn't quite done the trick, soda companies took a different tack. They announced a new and improved voluntary school policy, this time negotiated with the Clinton Foundation (the former president has made childhood obesity one of his post-presidency causes) and the American Heart Association (AHA).[22] While the nutrition standards are marginally better, they still allow diet soda, sports drinks, and other unhealthy beverages in high schools. But what didn't change is that the policy is still completely voluntary and lacking any accountability. While industry did this time promise to "compile the percentage of schools in compliance" and make this information publicly available beginning in August 2007, how the companies will determine compliance is a mystery. Moreover, it's up to the schools to renegotiate their contracts. But what if they don't?

I was particularly incensed by this move because for several months prior, I had been part of a team of ten attorneys and public health groups who were in private negotiation with lawyers from the American Beverage Association, Coca-Cola, and PepsiCo. From these meetings—operating under the threat of litigation being planned in Massachusetts—we got close to an agreement that was oddly similar to the one announced with Bill Clinton. Apparently, Coke and Pepsi were shopping around for the best PR opportunity; it looks much better to have a former president at your side than a bunch of lawyers. What a brilliant strategy by the soda companies, telling us they were bargaining in good faith, all the while planning another deal. Do we really need any more evidence that food and beverage companies cannot be trusted?

The main purpose in bringing a lawsuit is to ensure that the companies are held accountable to the outcome, whether by court decision or settlement agreement. Similarly, the current effort in state legislatures all over the nation to pass bills to rid schools of unhealthy drinks (which, as we will see, Coke and Pepsi lobby against vociferously) would *require* actual policy change. But industry prefers self-regulation, an unenforceable system that has already proven to be a dismal failure. Since the soda companies' first PR stunt didn't make their problems go away, Coke and Pepsi just came up with a better idea. But is Bill Clinton going to visit every school in the nation to ensure that this policy is implemented? In the meantime, the announcement might quell ongoing grassroots efforts, state legislation, and other, enforceable policies. Indeed, in several states where school nutrition bills were pending at the time of the announcement, the local AHA advocate was told that she could no longer support such legislation as a result of the deal forged at the national level.[23]

This, in a nutshell, is what is so dangerous about the efforts of corporations to position themselves as responsible citizens committed to upholding the public's best interests: such maneuvers can be extremely effective at lulling policy makers, advocates, and the general public into a false sense of security. Corporations, we are reassured, are taking care of the problem; public participation in the policymaking process is no longer required.

But food corporations cannot be trusted to protect the public's health. Accepting this truth will go a long way to a deeper understanding of how companies are responding to criticism and should provide you with the healthy dose of skepticism you will need to evaluate their claims. Once you realize that every move a food company makes is designed to protect its bottom line, you can then more clearly recognize corporate behavior and not let it fool you.

Personal Responsibility, Energy Balance, and Other Distractions

We believe this is all about energy balance.[1]
—Shelly Rosen, director of McDonald's "Eat Smart, Be Active" program

Food companies are in a quandary. On the one hand, if they acknowledge rocketing rates of diabetes, heart disease, and other diet-related maladies, they embroil themselves in a public relations nightmare: talking about their own culpability in creating these problems. On the other hand, plausible denial is extremely risky, given the overwhelming scientific evidence.

So, many food corporations, trade associations, and industry front groups are adopting an intermediary approach: admitting there's a problem but laying the blame elsewhere—with the individual. Call it the "personal responsibility" strategy. This line of reasoning goes like this: it's up to each individual to make "better" choices at supermarkets and restaurants. More importantly, it's each person's duty to make positive lifestyle changes, such as exercising more. Consumers who are having difficulty figuring out the "right" options for healthier living are simply in need of "better education"—which food marketers and PR mavens are happy to supply, but of course only in the most corporate-friendly ways.

The Mother of All Distractions: Personal Responsibility

The food industry's personal responsibility mantra has been invoked as a familiar rationale for less government action on a variety of social issues. For example, the Personal Responsibility and Work Opportunity Reconciliation Act of 1996 was President Clinton's attempt to "reform" the welfare system by scaling back federal funding for its various "safety net" programs. In the context of obesity, food makers have rallied behind the Personal Responsibility in Consumption Act, a federal bill that would ban obesity-related lawsuits. In proposing the bill, Representative Ric Keller (R-FL) explains that "[w]e need to get back to the principles of personal responsibility and away from the culture where everybody plays the victim."[2] Steven Anderson, CEO of the National Restaurant Association, invokes similar rhetoric in support of the legislation. "Restaurants," says Anderson, "should not be blamed for issues of personal responsibility and freedom of choice."[3]

Connecting the concepts of personal responsibility and freedom of choice is the key tactic of the Center for Consumer

Freedom (CCF), the food industry's master front group and spin-maker. Its mission is to "promote personal responsibility and protect consumer choices."[4] Because CCF's main strategy is to deny the problem of obesity altogether, it is less concerned with blaming the victim than other industry groups. Rather, CCF is more invested in depicting government regulation as a threat to the very notion of personal responsibility.

One goal of this approach is to frame the issue in starkly black-and-white terms: people, CCF insists, are simply wrong to blame others for their own problems.

But of course it's not that simple. Those of us who advocate policy-based solutions do not believe that individual behavior is irrelevant. I certainly don't. (But that doesn't stop CCF from claiming that I'm the kind of writer whose "words spell trouble for personal responsibility," in the "biography" the group created for me.[5]) Rather, we are suggesting that government has an important role to play in helping people make better, more informed choices and lead healthier lives.

To understand how to respond to the personal responsibility argument, let's examine the myths associated with this line of reasoning.

Myth: *People know that certain foods are unhealthy*

The argument that people should assume personal responsibility for their food choices presupposes that everyone has equal access to the information needed to make decisions intelligently. CCF likes to drive home this point with

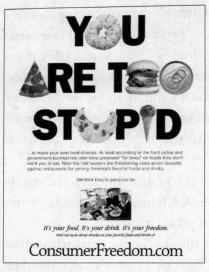

Center for Consumer Freedom Ad

bumper sticker slogans like "You are too stupid . . . to make your own food choices."[6] Such campaigns are designed to spew venom at the so-called food police (i.e., those advocating government regulation), deriding them for denying you, wise consumer, the capacity to make adult choices about foods you know very well might be bad for you. But this argument is both disingenuous and hypocritical.

It is certainly true that in recent years more information has become available about the health consequences of eating the standard American diet, which consists largely of high-fat animal products and a wide assortment of highly processed, nutritionally deficient foods. Books such as Eric Schlosser's *Fast Food Nation* (along with the movie version) and documentary films like Morgan Spurlock's *Super Size Me*, for example, have drawn attention to the myriad ills (personal and social) to which fast-food chains like McDonald's have contributed. But despite the increased media attention, not everyone fully understands the scope of the food industry's role in creating such problems. And how could they, given that so much of the relevant information is distorted or kept hidden by food manufacturers and government agencies alike? For example, restaurant chains are refusing to provide even with the most basic nutrition information to help people exercise more personal responsibility. There are numerous examples of how food-industry lobbyists control and manipulate the discourse on food and food policy.

Myth: People can simply choose to eat healthy foods

An important tenet of the food industry's personal responsibility argument is that options for "healthier" eating are virtually limitless, especially since food companies are now hard at work churning out more and more "alternatives" just waiting to be gobbled up. Really, it's all up to you. As the Grocery Manufacturers Association (GMA) self-righteously inveighs: "Providing a wide variety of nutritious foods and beverages, and helping parents make the right choices for their families, is our industry's top priority."[7] Setting aside for now the question of whether it's even true that industry is providing healthier food, the sobering reality is that most people do not have access to truly healthy foods, such as fresh fruits and vegetables. I am fortunate to live in northern California, where fresh, seasonal produce is available throughout the year. My home in Oakland is within easy walking distance to one large grocery chain, two small local stores that sell healthy food, and a weekly farmers' market. I also own a car, which means I can drive to a nearby large natural-foods store when I need to.

Regrettably, such a situation is the exception rather than the rule for most people in this country. In fact, only a few miles from my home in every direction are neighborhoods without a farmers' market or even a full-service grocery store. Here many people are dependent on unreliable public transportation, making the corner liquor store or mini-mart—where nourishment options range from Coke to Fritos—the only realistic food-shopping venue.

Even for people who can shop in large supermarkets, access to genuinely healthy food remains limited. Most chains don't sell a wide variety of natural whole grains, and their "fresh" fruits or vegetables are often sterile, tasteless, pesticide-soaked, and nutritionally challenged. And no wonder, since the year-round produce in large chains is cultivated for extended shelf life, portability, and cosmetic uniformity, traits that benefit the seller—not the buyer. That's why the tomatoes taste like cardboard and the fruit is rock-hard. And while it's true that large "natural food" retailers like Whole Foods are opening more stores, the products at such high-end markets are unaffordable for most people. (Whole Foods' sometime nickname, "Whole Paycheck," is well earned.)

Faced with these "choices," it's understandable why people turn to highly processed, inexpensive foods—often, they're the only game in town. We cannot talk about people taking personal responsibility for their food choices without an honest discussion about the lack of access to affordable, truly healthy food.

Myth: Marketing has little impact on food choices

What also often gets lost in the personal responsibility discussion is the fact that the food industry spend upwards of $36 billion annually to market its products. The food business is extremely competitive. While most of us like to think we're immune to advertising, the truth is that corporations do not keep spending that kind of cash without expecting a handsome return on their investment.

The reality is that we are all influenced by advertising, whether we know it or not, or whether we care to admit it or not. There are volumes written on this topic.[8] Isn't it amazing that food companies spend so much money trying to convince you to consume endless amounts of their unhealthy products and then turn right around and blame you for succumbing to that very same marketing?

Unfortunately, counterstrategies such as government-sponsored "5 a Day" programs—which encourage eating fruits and vegetables—simply cannot compete. Such poorly funded efforts to promote diets based on the right kinds of food are essentially squelched by savvy, well-financed corporate marketing aimed at getting people to eat more and more of the wrong kinds.

Myth: Parents can just say no to their kids

In the public debate over childhood obesity, personal responsibility polemicists like to give parents a bad rap. Since it's rather difficult for food companies to hold young children accountable for their poor food decisions, blaming their parents is a convenient workaround. Common refrains in this context include: "Children don't drive themselves to the fast-food joints"; "Parents just need to turn off the television"; and the ever-popular "Parents should set a better example."

Of course parents have a critical role to play in teaching their children good eating habits and in modeling that behavior. However, we also cannot ignore the fact that food corporations spend roughly $12 billion a year on marketing designed to get children to pester their parents for junk food—doing an end run around parents' authority over their kids' dietary choices in the process. (For more on this tactic and ways to respond to it, see Chapter 11.)

They're Not Holding a Gun to Your Head (but Almost)

An overarching theme of industry's personal responsibility argument goes something like this: "Food companies aren't holding a gun to anyone's head." Technically, this is of course true, but the rhetoric rings hollow upon closer inspection. Brandishing a firearm isn't the only way to get someone to behave in a way that goes against her own best interests. Indeed, food marketers have discovered countless other subtler, but nevertheless highly effective, strategies for achieving the same end.

Let's imagine we're astronauts who have just landed on an uninhabited planet. Our mission is to create a society where people get sick from eating too much of the wrong kinds of food. How would we go about doing this? Well, first we would make all of the least healthy foods cheap, readily available, and convenient to prepare and eat. Next, we would concoct mysterious chemical ingredients in laboratories to ensure that the food is exceptionally tasty in ways that are irreproducible by mortal home chefs. Then we would market the hell out of these foods, in every form of media available. We would use highly sophisticated advertising techniques, including subliminal messages, in an effort to make these products even more alluring—so irresistible, in fact, that people would want to consume them frequently and in large quantities, thus guaranteeing addictive tendencies. We would also make sure that all of the healthiest foods were expensive and inaccessible, and thought of as boring, unappealing, and elitist. Further, we would turn cooking into a lost art reserved only for highly trained professionals and television entertainment. Finally, our little band of interplanetary invaders would hijack the scientific process, suppress the truth about good nutrition, and deprive government programs of adequate funding to promote healthy eating. This is exactly the situation we have today.

The point of this exercise is not to accuse food corporations of engaging in an evil conspiracy to make people sick. Rather, it is to illustrate that various economic, political, and social processes are operating beyond the control of most individuals, restricting their access to healthy foods and constraining their ability to make informed dietary choices. While there may be no proverbial smoking gun, for many people, society is essentially arranged such that there might as well be.

Exercise and Energy Balance:
The Excuses that Keep on Giving

A variation on the personal responsibility theme is this: it's time Americans got off their lazy duffs. Food companies, trade associations, and industry front groups love to portray lack of exercise as the "true cause" of (and hence the solution to) the obesity epidemic. This is, of course, a great way to deflect blame while changing the subject. For example, in responding to pressure to get soda out of schools, the American Beverage Association indicts our couch potato culture with this ready quip: "It's about the Couch, Not the Can."[9] Other times, the goal is to position obesity as being too complex to be reduced to a single "solution" (e.g., food), as reflected in this line from the GMA: "Effective solutions to obesity must take a comprehensive approach, incorporating sound nutrition, increased physical activity, consumer and parent education, and community support."[10]

For the Center for Consumer Freedom, the objectives are more brazen still. Indeed, CCF has gone so far as to advance two seemingly contradictory positions: one, that lack of exercise is the principal cause of obesity, and two, that there is, in fact, no obesity epidemic. Apparently, logical inconsistency of argument poses no barrier to deployment. For example, in a letter published in the *Boston Globe* (which sadly neglected to reveal the organization's industry ties), CCF's Dan Mindus had little compunction about criticizing a Harvard University study on weight and health: "What Americans need is a healthy dose of exercise, not another needless and unfounded lecture about their weight."[11] (That there may be some scientific connection between weight and exercise is, again, of no consequence to CCF's illogical framing.) Mindus's remark illustrates how the exercise argument is used, like other subroutines in the personal responsibility blame game, to deflect attention away from an industry-created public health problem, distort scientific claims, and maintain the focus on individual behavior change.

I try to listen very closely to the rhetoric that food company executives and trade-group representatives use. I'm no fan of conspiracy theories, but when I begin to notice the repeated use of certain catchphrases and sound bites by different corporate representatives, I can't help wondering if they've called a meeting to get everyone on message. In

2003, industry's increasingly habitual use of the term "energy balance" as code for the real solution to the obesity problem emerged on my radar screen. By 2004, the phrase was virtually ubiquitous. Here are just a few of the numerous ways it's been wielded by food-industry representatives: (1) "We believe this [obesity] is all about energy balance" (Shelly Rosen, McDonald's),[12] (2) "Like most experts in the health field, I believe that the ultimate solution to the obesity problem is energy balance" (Susan Finn, American Council for Fitness and Nutrition),[13] (3) "We believe, as do many nutrition experts, that solving the obesity problem is about maintaining a healthy lifestyle and achieving the proper energy balance" (Alison Kretser, Grocery Manufacturers Association).[14]

In the context of the obesity problem, the scientific-sounding term "energy balance" aims to neutralize what might otherwise be a highly politically charged discussion about the role of food and nutrition policy. Here's how food and beverage giant PepsiCo deploys this mollifying aim:

> Energy balance: it's really quite simple. It's a balance between what we eat and what we do. Another way to think of it: energy in from food, and energy out from activity. When we eat, our bodies take in calories and turn them into energy.[15]

Linda Bacon, a nutrition and physiology expert with the University of California, Davis, says the energy balance concept, as utilized by food marketers like PepsiCo, is overly simplistic at best:

This is more confusing than it appears on the surface. We can't control energy balance. For example, we may exercise to burn extra calories, but our body may decide that losing weight is unhealthy for us and get conservative in other ways so that you stay in energy balance, despite increasing activity. In other words, gaining/losing weight is a lot more confusing than just cutting calories or exercising, and some of this is beyond our control.[16]

Of course, food sellers are not about to let such conceptual complexities stand in the way of using objective-sounding terms like *energy balance* in their campaign to enshrine individual lifestyle change as *the* solution to the obesity crisis.

Funding the distractions: exercise philanthropy

In playing the "exercise" card, food companies have yet another opportunity to position themselves as "part of the solution." A time-honored corporate PR tactic is to use philanthropy to deflect critics. Most of the major food companies are donating money or otherwise funding programs related to exercise, especially where children might benefit. In doing so, companies are seeking maximum positive PR effect. The ways that industry funds physical activity generally fall into the following categories: (1) Web-based education, sponsored by one or more companies; (2) in-school programs; (3) joint programs with public entities (universities or government); (4) donations to nonprofits and/or communities. The purpose is almost always the same: to gain positive PR while deflecting criticism.

Most of the time, it's obvious that the program has corporate sponsorship. Other times, you have to dig a little to find out. But in all of the examples I found, the information is available on the program Web sites, so it's not hidden if you know where to look. Where it's less obvious, there are red flags, including the use of key catchphrases such as "energy balance" and "healthy lifestyles." (For a guide to such philanthropic programs, see Appendix 2.)

Branded playgrounds

In a demonstration of infinite corporate chutzpah, PepsiCo is funding branded playgrounds for kids. In November 2005, the company opened a playground in a Washington, D.C. preschool, the first of thirteen planned sites.[17] Brock Leach, PepsiCo's chief innovation officer, explained that funding playgrounds is "all about moving more, helping kids move more."[18]

Never mind that the equipment bears the company's "Smart Spot" logo, which is also placed on food packaging to "help" consumers make "healthier" food choices among PepsiCo's products (including such "smart" choices as Diet Pepsi and Baked Lays). The cost of the playground is about $850,000. Even multiplying that by the thirteen sites, the figure pales in comparison to the company's revenues of more than $32 billion in 2005 alone.[19] How about donating the money quietly to community groups so they can decide what colors to use and which messages to place on the equipment, if any? The PR goal is clear, as corporate spokesman Mark Dollins admits: "Smart Spot is targeted to moms, not kids. We want moms to see us as on their side."[20] Of course they do; what better way to ensure that "moms" continue to purchase the company's ubiquitous salty snacks and sugary drinks in the wake of a childhood obesity crisis? No problem here, moms, we got your kids covered with a big green slide.

Clowning around

Never one to miss out on a good PR bandwagon, McDonald's is also encouraging kids to get fit. With the fast-food king's notorious child-themed marketing increasingly under attack by advocates, McDonald's is in dire need of spin control. So, what better way to clean up your image (rather than your act) than to turn the corporate mascot into a marketing machine for exercise? It's a win-win strategy. McDonald's gains another excuse to market its brand and spread goodwill while promoting a politically safe and upbeat message.

That explains why, in January 2005, McDonald's Chief Creative Officer Marlena Peleo-Lazar told a government panel concerned with food marketing to children (whose members needed to be won over) that Ronald McDonald had morphed from "chief happiness officer" into an "ambassador for an active, balanced lifestyle" and was visiting elementary schools to tout exercise.[21]

That's not all. In June 2005, the marketing machine decided it was time for Ronald to *look* more active if he was truly going to *be* active. So, after forty-two years, the mascot traded in his trademark yellow jumpsuit for sportier garb. While a television commercial was planned to unveil the refurbished mascot, the press was first duly alerted for maximum PR effect. The result was an avalanche of news stories appearing in both print and broadcast media, days before the commercial even aired. Newspapers ran with headlines such as, "Ronald McDonald Gets Extreme

Makeover,"[22] "McDonald's Gives Ronald Jock Makeover to Fit with Healthier Menu,"[23] "Ronald McJock? McDonald's Gives Mascot Sporty New Look."[24] Not all reporters were fooled, though. Reuters news service said, "The reincarnated Ronald is part of McDonald's aggressive effort to deflect widespread media criticism of its food as unhealthy and fattening."[25]

But wait, there's more. Just in case the PR train might be slowing down, McDonald's marketing team revved it up again in fall 2005 with a new program called Active Achievers, which "delivers educational messages to students about nutrition, and balance between eating right and staying active."[26] (Just what we need: the top purveyor of burgers, shakes, and fries "educating" kids about nutrition.) As if that weren't enough, McDonald's also announced in the fall of 2005 a program called "Passport to Play," which was distributed to thirty-one thousand schools and seven million children, designed to "motivate children to be more active in unique and fun ways during grade school physical education classes."[27]

Psychologist Susan Linn, author of *Consuming Kids* and cofounder of the Campaign for a Commercial-Free Childhood, says McDonald's has no place in school: "This is just another marketing ploy. The notion that children need Ronald McDonald to get them to enjoy exercise is bogus. Given the opportunity, kids naturally like to be active."[28]

But such minor details are of no concern to a major marketing machine like McDonald's. If parents think that Ronald is helping kids get more active, that positive feeling might spill over into food purchases, thereby minimizing any risk of decreased sales due to negative PR about the company's unhealthy food. But if McDonald's really cared about changing kids' behavior, wouldn't it make more sense for the company to simply stop getting kids hooked on Happy Meals with toys and other promotions that don't have anything to do with food?

McDONALD'S AND EXERCISE PROMOTION

Announces Global Advisory Council on Balanced Lifestyles	May 2003
Announces "Balanced Lifestyles Platform" (Partnership with fitness guru Bob Greene)	April 2004
Launches New Worldwide Balanced, Active Lifestyles Public Awareness Campaign	March 2005
Ronald McDonald Gets an Extreme Makeover	June 2005
Active Achievers and Passport to Play programs	September 2005

Education, Brought to You by Coke

In the imagination of food companies and their lobbyists, education ranks right up there with exercise as a key component of the personal responsibility solution. Individuals, the argument goes, need to be better educated, so that they can make dietary decisions that are right for them based on their personal energy needs and health concerns. The claim that education "empowers" people to make the right product choices is a thinly veiled jab at nutrition advocates, who are chastised as "food cops" bent on taking away the rights of consumers—even children—to freely decide which foods are best for them.

Of course, when food companies speak of education, they don't just mean any old education, but rather the kind that *they* provide. The goal is to retain complete control over the information that people need to make dietary decisions. One of the more insidious manifestations of this strategy is how corporations are increasingly providing health education materials to schools. It's a rather brilliant PR move, since it allows food makers to continue targeting the lucrative kid market where they remain a captive audience in an authoritative setting.

For most cash-strapped public schools, the prospect of donated educational materials, even those plastered with corporate logos, is irresistible. In addition to McDonald's, soda companies are also targeting schools with their own "get healthy" messaging. For example, Coca-Cola lavished $4 million in the fall of 2005 on an educational program called "Live It!" developed for 8,500 public middle schools. The weeklong program featured videos in which cyclist Lance Armstrong and other famous sports figures encouraged children to be active.[29] Coke's lesson plan, which reached some two million students nationwide, contained some nutrition tips, but it made no mention of beverage consumption. For example, the program vacuously "emphasizes nutritious alternatives, such as fruits and vegetables, when making choices for lunch in the cafeteria."[30] Not to be outdone, rival soda maker PepsiCo came up with its own package of "forward-thinking" education materials in the fall of 2005. Pepsi's "Balance First" fitness program was initially aimed at some three million elementary school students, and it eventually made its way to all of the nation's 15,000 middle schools.

The developers of the Coca-Cola and PepsiCo fitness

programs apparently saw no irony in the fact that these companies also peddle unhealthy beverages in these same educational institutions. In their eyes, trusting corporations that make money selling flavored sugar water to teach children about good nutrition is a no-brainer; that's what responsible corporate citizenship is all about.

The disingenuousness of this approach to health education was revealed in the July 2005 edition of *PR Week*, which tracks the major players in the public relations industry. The magazine reported that "Coca-Cola will work with [mega PR firm] Weber Shandwick this fall to promote its new, seemingly selfless, Live It! children's fitness campaign in schools across the country." The PR firm will "focus on generating local publicity for schools that participate in the weeklong program."[31] But if Coca-Cola really cared about kids, why would the company need to spend so much money on public relations to generate media attention for its "seemingly selfless" program?

Live It! followed on the heels of Coke's Step With It! curriculum, which reached more than one million kids aged ten to fourteen in 2005. According to Widmeyer Communications, another major PR company hired by Coke, the challenge was to "demonstrate to the public that the [Coca-Cola] Company was committed to being a part of the solution, not the problem" in the face of increasing criticism from public-interest groups and grassroots movements, which are working to kick Coke out of schools in the wake of mounting scientific evidence linking childhood obesity to high rates of soda consumption.[32] Quite a challenge indeed.

When it comes to educating our children about good nutrition, we can surely find better pedagogical tools than companies whose principal purpose is to generate revenue from the sale of unhealthy food and drink. While these corporations would have you believe they're helping poor schools with much-needed resources, reliable alternatives abound for nutrition curricula and other school-based information for improving children's health. (See Appendix 6.)

PEPSICO'S EDUCATIONAL PROGRAMS

- Balance First (in-school curriculum)
- Get Active Stay Active (part of President's Challenge)
- Get Kids in Action (Gatorade sponsored)
- Kidnetic.com (with numerous other food companies)
- P.E. 4 Life (Gatorade sponsored)
- S.M.A.R.T. Living (part of Smart Spot "seal" program)
- America on the Move (main sponsor, with others)

Responding to the Education Argument

Promoting education as a catch-all solution to obesity accomplishes many of the same corporate objectives as other tactics in the personal responsibility arsenal, and all in the guise of a seemingly value-neutral and eminently reasonable concept. Who, after all, would argue that people shouldn't be more educated? Once again, the picture is not as black-and-white as industry would have it appear. Underlying the oversimplified rhetoric are several myths that can help you respond to this corporate magic wand solution.

Myth: Policy solutions would replace education

Of course, educating people about good nutrition is important.

Nobody is denying that. Indeed, I think we need to improve the quality of nutrition education, unfiltered through corporate interests. However, nutrition education alone is insufficient to address the diet-related public health crisis in the country today. The basic philosophy of the nutrition profession, the idea that a combination of individual counseling and "social marketing" (mass education) will promote healthy eating behavior, has already proven inadequate, to say the least. Just talk to any dietitian about how hard it is to get clients to change their behavior. The problem is that once people are "educated," they return to the real world, where unhealthy foods abound and affordable access to genuinely healthy alternatives is lacking. What we need are policies that don't constantly undermine efforts to educate people about proper nutrition; that is, by making healthy foods affordable and widely available.

Myth: Maintaining the status quo is education

A variation of the food industry's education-will-save-us argument goes something like this: consumers must be guaranteed access to the full array of food options currently on the market. This will ensure that people (especially children) have the freedom to "learn" about and "choose" those products that are best for them. This hands-off approach represents the best kind of food-related "education." The suggestion that food choices (in schools, for example) should be restricted in any way is just more meddling by the food police. Here's how Alison Kretser, senior director of scientific and nutrition policy for the Grocery Manufacturers Association, put it in her testimony against a Maryland bill aimed at curtailing the

sale of junk food in public schools: "Restrictions do not educate. It is through education—both nutrition and physical—
that we will empower students to adopt a healthy lifestyle that
meets their own needs and allows them to enjoy their favorite
foods as part of a balanced diet."[33]

And how exactly does maintaining the status quo, which is
so heavily weighted toward unhealthy options, further "education"? While it may be true that restricting junk foods
could make them more desirable, especially to children, this
is no excuse for schools to give junk food an educational
stamp of approval. After all, how do we expect children to
learn about health and nutrition in the classroom only to have
those lessons undermined by the sale of unhealthy food just
steps away in the cafeteria (not to mention hallway vending
machines, canteens, etc.)? Proponents of the education
model of reform would rather we close our eyes to this
obvious contradiction by conducting business as usual.

Myth: Education means freedom to eat crap

Of course, when food lobbyists proclaim education as the
answer, they have in mind a very specific type of education—
the kind that perpetuates overconsumption of their unhealthy
products, and leaves big corporations firmly in charge of the
information we receive about nutrition and good health. The
GMA's Alison Kretser admonished us that education is
needed so that children are free to "adopt a healthy lifestyle
that meets their own needs" and "enjoy their favorite foods."

What Kretser is effectively saying is that it's up to you,
kids, to figure out which of your "favorite" (industry code

for "junk") foods best fit you and your "healthy lifestyle."
(When did kids start having "lifestyles" instead of a life?) The
genius of this rhetoric is that it sanctions the status quo of
junk food marketing run amok, while making food manufacturers appear to be caring corporate citizens who are
deeply concerned about "education" and the "freedom" to
acquire it.

The Blame Game

The corporate strategies discussed in this chapter all boil
down to this blunt message: it's all your fault. It's up to each
individual to solve the problem of poor health in the United
States. You have made certain choices about how you eat,
move, and inform yourself, and it's up to you to make different decisions to improve your physical condition.

Eerily, this is a tune we've heard before. I asked Richard
Daynard, professor at Northeastern University School of Law
and veteran of the tobacco wars, about how cigarette companies used "personal responsibility" as a strategy. He said the
concept was "one of the leading defenses that the tobacco
industry used both in the courtroom and in the court of
public opinion." He continued:

> Basically, the personal responsibility argument was that
> anybody who is stupid enough to use their products
> and gullible enough to believe the companies when
> they said their products don't cause lung cancer and
> other diseases, deserve to get those diseases. That's
> what it boils down to when you unpack it: that the
> companies are blaming you. Saying that you really have

to be stupid to buy our product was a great way to defend the lawsuits, but not a great strategy for selling cigarettes. They tried to avoid actually coming out and saying that, but they got very close.[34]

It's no accident that corporations use similar strategies across issues; they know what works in the minds of the public. Playing on traditional American notions of "rugged individualism," the personal responsibility argument conveniently deflects attention away from the manufacturing and marketing of unhealthy food by placing the onus for change solely on the shoulders of individual consumers. Moreover, it allows food makers to dismiss calls for government regulation and instead position themselves as "responsible corporate citizens" whose products and educational services constitute an important "part of the solution."

Toward a Broader Model of Change

One of the main goals of nutrition policy should be to shift the focus from individual blame to a broader societal outlook. As I mentioned before, for decades, nutritionists have focused on an education-based model for behavioral change. However, it has become painfully clear that education alone does not work. A new movement is taking hold aimed at policy changes to help people make better decisions about diet and health. The idea is for healthy eating to be the default instead of constantly being the more challenging way to live.

The food industry understands this new direction in food policy well and is threatened by it. That's why it's intent on holding individuals alone responsible for their own fate. We must not, however, allow corporations to frame the debate for us. We can acknowledge the importance of personal responsibility, but we must also demand a society designed to support individual behavior change. The question must not simply be, "How can individuals take better care of themselves?" We must also ask, "How can society—including major institutional players such as government and corporations—make it easier for people to live healthy lives?"

3

Freedom from Choice:
Distortions of
All-American Values

Our offensive strategy is to shoot the messenger. Given the activists' plans to alarm beyond all reason, we've got to attack their credibility as spokespersons.[1]

—Richard Berman, director of the industry front group
Center for Consumer Freedom

When you think of organizations like the American Medical Association (AMA), the American Corn Growers Association, the Harvard School of Public Health, or the U.S. Centers for Disease Control and Prevention, do the words "radical activists" immediately spring to mind? They would if you saw the world through the eyes of an industry front group whose mission is to discredit any group that might interfere with corporate profits.

Outsourcing the Dirty Work

In order to protect their squeaky-clean reputations, individual food companies tend to outsource the grittier public relations work to trade associations and industry front groups. One organization has distinguished itself in this sphere: the Center for Consumer Freedom (CCF). In almost Orwellian fashion, CCF conceals its real motivations, biases, and objectives behind a faux-populist name. Far from representing "consumers," the group is in fact a lobby for the restaurant, food, beverage, alcohol, and tobacco industries. Headed by Richard (aka Rick) Berman, a notorious tobacco lobbyist, CCF began its life under an equally innocuous-sounding moniker, the "Guest Choice Network"—which represented the hospitality industry up until 2002—courtesy of a $600,000 grant from Phillip Morris.[2] In total, the tobacco giant has lavished close to $3 million on Berman's cause,[3] which should give you a good idea of its philosophical underpinnings. It's no surprise, then, that CCF boasts a well-financed and highly sophisticated media tool kit, which includes regular press releases, advertising campaigns, op-ed articles, letters to the editor, television appearances, and numerous Web sites.

In 2005, industry representatives (who spoke only on the condition that they not be identified) revealed to the *Washington Post* that by keeping its corporate sponsors anonymous, CCF "can be more vociferous, provocative, and irreverent in its criticisms than a trade association." CCF director Rick Berman cheerfully confirmed that organizations like his are poised to dabble in edgier PR, a tactic that provides individual corporations safe shelter: "There's no doubt about that. Most trade associations try to insulate individual companies and brand names from cutting-edge rhetoric."[4] Thus, trade associations and front groups are at liberty to play the "bad cops" to, say, Kraft's and PepsiCo's "good cops."

Berman's group specializes in the kind of no-holds-barred intimidation tactics pioneered by Big Tobacco. I got to experience this myself twice in a recent two-year period, when within days of my publishing op-ed articles critical of Big Food, I received letters from CCF requesting the financial records of my nonprofit organization, the Center for Informed Food Choices. Because such requests legally require a response, CCF succeeded in wasting my time and (quite meager) resources; they did not, however, deter me from continuing to tell the truth about industry practices. CCF has also forced larger organizations such as the Physicians Committee for Responsible Medicine (PCRM) to defend themselves against distortions and outright lies. Among other allegations, CCF has repeatedly accused PCRM of having been "censured" by the AMA, a charge that PCRM president Neal Barnard, a lifetime member, dismisses as "patently untrue."[5]

Dismantling the Attack Dog Rhetoric

While most food lobbyists rely on the rhetoric of "personal responsibility" to blame the obesity problem on the failure of individuals to behave sensibly, CCF, in contrast, chooses to deny the problem altogether. Their position is to "defend" the very notion of personal responsibility by tying it closely to the all-American values of choice, freedom, and rugged individualism. Against whom do these values need to be defended? The food police, militant radicals, and Big Brother government bureaucrats who want to keep you from enjoying your God-given right to Big Macs, Marlboros, and Budweiser.

Of course CCF didn't invent this notion of individualism. It pervades society—in weight-loss programs, diet-advice books, and other educational messages. The trouble is, such narrow reasoning conveniently sidesteps the many complex variables that influence behavior, such as upbringing and psychology, not to mention relentless exposure to ubiquitous food marketing. By keeping the focus on the independent consumer, CCF is able to deflect criticism of food corporations' products and practices, leaving industry firmly in control of the policy discourse.

Us vs. Them

One of CCF's favorite strategies is to align the interests of food companies with those of consumers. It portrays these two "allied" groups as the besieged "victims" of government regulators, nonprofits, parents, and other food-industry critics who make up the burgeoning ranks of the "food police." The narrative is familiar: food corporations are on your side, dear consumer; we care about you; we're looking out for you. We're providing you with many wonderful food and beverage choices, and we want to make sure that you'll continue to be able to enjoy them. Those bad guys—the people working to impose regulations on food sellers and file lawsuits against them—they think they know what is best for you, but they don't. We do, however; so believe us, not them.

Together we can beat back those big, bad food police and safeguard the American way of life!

All-American food, good; healthy food, bad

What does CCF mean, exactly, by "consumer freedom"? Let's see what they have to say: "Consumer freedom is the right of adults and parents to choose what they eat, drink, and how they enjoy themselves. Defending enjoyment is what we're all about!"[6] "Defending enjoyment," who could argue with that? As if enjoyment needs defending. Does it appear to you that enjoyment is really under serious threat in this country? The implication, of course, is that the interests of the people who advocate for sound nutrition policy are somehow diametrically opposed to everyone else's, and that anyone concerned about good nutrition is a killjoy with no interest in enjoying food. This taps into the popular view that cheeseburgers, fries, shakes, soda, and other standard junk foods are as American as apple pie, while eating healthfully is elitist, dull, and rather sappy.

Children in the shadow of the big, bad food police

A related salvo in CCF's free-to-choose argument is the notion that nutrition advocates and other food-industry critics are infantilizing people when they give dietary advice. CCF produced a television commercial showing people trying to enjoy all-American pleasures such as ice cream, hot dogs, and beer, only to be foiled by a hand that swoops down and commandeers the offending items before they can reach the salivating palates. A friendly voice-over inveighs: "Everywhere you turn, someone's telling us what we can't eat. It's getting harder just to enjoy a beer on a night out. Do you always feel like you're being told what to do? Find out who is driving the food police at ConsumerFreedom.com."[7] What true, red-blooded American could resist this call for a life of adult dietary independence, free from Big Brother's long, dark shadow of paternalistic surveillance and control? Of course, this is just a silly distraction from the very real health problems advocates are talking about.

"RADICAL" ORGANIZATIONS ATTACKED BY CCF (A VERY PARTIAL LIST)[8]

Action on Smoking and Health
American Medical Association
American Corn Growers Association
Center for Food Safety
Center for Science in the Public Interest
Consumer Federation of America
Earth Island Institute
Friends of the Earth
Harvard School of Public Health
Mothers Against Drunk Driving
National Association of High School Principals
Organic Consumers Association
Physicians' Committee for Responsible Medicine
U.S. Centers for Disease Control and Prevention

Shooting the Messenger: A Convenient Misdirect

When it comes to inciting people to cower in fear of the food police, directing attention away from the substantive issues, and keeping the focus on the messenger instead of the message, CCF has few scruples. Any person or advocacy group that has the temerity to suggest that the government do its job and protect the public from harm inflicted by deceitful corporations is fair game for its hit list. For example, CCF has created a Web site known as CSPIscam, whose sole purpose is to discredit and defame one of the nation's leading nutrition advocacy organizations, the Center for Science in the Public Interest (CSPI). The site insists that the nonprofit "and its founder, Michael F. Jacobson, are not as nice, sweet, and unbiased as CSPI's name might imply. The group routinely uses scare tactics justified by 'junk science' and media theatrics as part of their ceaseless campaign for government regulation of your personal food choices."[9]

In dismissing CSPI's work as media driven and reliant upon "junk science" (a favorite derisive term for any research that inconveniently goes against corporate interests), CCF's aim is to scare people into believing that the group is trying to take away their God-given right to eat whatever they want. I have been closely following CSPI for many years, and have found that, unlike some other groups, CSPI backs up every claim it makes and is actually quite cautious about its scientific conclusions. Does CSPI use the media effectively? Absolutely. But that makes it neither a devotee of "media theatrics" nor out to usurp anyone's food choices. It is simply asking the government to protect the American people from overexposure to food makers' unhealthy products.

Those militant nutritionists and their radical agendas

Here is how the Center for Consumer Freedom explains its mission:

The growing cabal of "food cops," health-care enforcers, militant activists, meddling bureaucrats, and violent radicals who think they know "what's best for you" are pushing against our basic freedoms. We're here to push back.[10]

An important objective of such rhetoric is to marginalize advocates and set them apart from mainstream America. What better way to do this than to use phrases such as "militant activists" and "violent radicals"? These labels are meant to conjure up caricatured images of 1960s-style activism, complete with flag burning, sex, drugs, and rock and roll. If we don't watch out, CCF insinuates, those crazy nutritionists might invade our homes and burn down our barbecues and ice cream makers in the name of public health! The truth is that nutrition advocates are among the most mainstream people you could ever know. They include doctors, nurses, dietitians, teachers, public health researchers, politicians, and other professionals—hardly a bunch of radical bomb throwers. I've never seen violence break out at any of their meetings. In fact, with this crowd, a heated discussion on the merits of the latest school vending machine policy is about as fierce as things are likely to get.

CCF has even developed a Web site called ActivistCash, which claims to "expose" the funding sources of various environmental and public health organizations. (Never mind that such information is already publicly available.)

Also on this site, you'll find a guide to the "key players" in nutrition advocacy. Among the people singled out is New York University nutrition professor Marion Nestle, who is described as "one of the country's most hysterical anti-food-industry fanatics," a food cop with "radical goals."[11] In truth, Nestle is one of the nation's most respected voices in nutrition policy, and has authored several authoritative books on the topic, including the highly acclaimed *Food Politics.* Major newspapers such as the *New York Times* routinely solicit Nestle's opinions on nutrition issues and publish her writings. CCF's name-calling is clearly designed to marginalize her viewpoints, which are often critical of the food industry. Nestle notes that CCF staffers have even gone so far as to stalk her at her lectures, in a frantic effort to appropriate material for their own propagandistic ends: "For a while, they were going to every talk I gave and quoting me out of context. I think their tactics are sleazy and any food company that supports them should be deeply ashamed."[12]

Personal and hidden agendas

Implicit in CCF's food cop rhetoric is the idea that people who advocate for eating a healthy diet are motivated by their own personal agendas, not the well-being of the public at large. In my bio on the ActivistCash Web site, CCF claims that I "attack all foods that don't fit [my] vegan agenda."[13] Actually, I don't have a vegan agenda, nor is it my goal to get everyone to eat the way I choose to. Naturally, the fact that I personally happen to eat a mostly vegan (devoid of animal products) diet does influence my advocacy work. I also think a diet that resembles my own would be optimal for most people. Does that mean that I have some secret plan to change everyone's eating habits to precisely match mine? Absolutely not.

The aim of CCF's "personal agenda" verbiage is to impugn advocates like me for acting on the basis of nefarious ulterior motives. I really hate to burst your bubble, CCF, but my resolve to support polices that promote the consumption of whole grains and fresh fruits and vegetables is based on decades of accepted nutrition science, not some twisted scheme to turn the world into Michele Simon clones. Indeed, "vegan" doesn't even accurately describe my position. Rather, I promote a *whole foods*, plant-based diet; there are plenty of vegan foods that don't fit that "agenda." But of course, CCF's smear rhetoric prefers to pass over a term like *whole foods*. The loaded word *vegan* is much better suited to its tar and feathering purposes, given its association, in some circles, with extremism and radical-fringe "lunacy" (thanks in large part to the hard work of CCF's well-oiled PR machine and others like it).

CCF maintains a long hit parade of food cops operating under supposed "hidden agendas." The front group is also fond of accusing pro-vegetarian organizations like the PCRM and the People for the Ethical Treatment of Animals (PETA) of hiding behind an animal rights platform. But here's the funny thing: these groups' agendas are not at all concealed— they *are* trying to protect animals, and they readily acknowledge this goal. PCRM and PETA just also happen to subscribe to the scientifically supported view that vegetarian diets are healthier than meat-centered ones. In CCF's myth-making, this scientific verdict on human nutrition is yet another pesky fact that it's prepared to ignore in the interest of smearing and marginalizing food-industry critics. Why engage in serious debate on the merits of the issue when name-calling is so much easier?

Fighting Back: Dispelling CCF's Myths

Once you understand the myths and assumptions behind CCF's worldview, it's rather easy to develop convincing counterarguments. Here a few ways to respond to the group's favorite rhetorical tropes.

When they say: Making the right food choices is about personal responsibility.

They assume: The status quo provides a full range of choices.

The fact that most people simply do not have access to healthy food options is of course of no concern to CCF. When CCF says *choice* it means those choices provided by industry. But why do corporations get to decide what "choices" we even have? The assumption here is that the *current* range of food options is ideal and that any attempt by advocates or government to alter or limit these choices is tyrannical. The truth is quite the opposite: in allowing corporations to unilaterally and undemocratically determine our food choices for us, we wholly abdicate our freedom to choose. Indeed, what we really have in our food environment is a grand illusion: freedom *from* choice masquerading as freedom *of* choice. The choice between Quarter Pounders, Oreos, Diet Mountain Dew, and Whole Grain Cocoa Puffs is really no choice at all.

When they say: Food cops want to restrict consumer choice.

They assume: Regulating corporate behavior equals restricting consumers.

It's important to distinguish between government control over individual rights and reasonable regulation of corporate behavior. CCF's use of "food cop" scare tactics is a devious attempt to equate the interests of corporations with those of individuals. This equation is of course patently false. The purpose of a corporation is to expand market share and make money for its shareholders. Any "threat" stemming from government oversight of that behavior will only be felt by bean counters concerned with the corporate bottom line, not the individual consumer, whose interests are, in fact, being safeguarded by such policies. For example, requiring fast-food companies to provide nutrition information on menus is not an infringement of personal freedoms, but rather a reasonable way to protect public health by ensuring that food corporations provide people with the information they need to make informed decisions about their products.

> **When they say:** We are defending your rights.
> **They assume:** There is an absolute right to eat whatever we want.

Legally and morally, no one can claim an absolute right to eat whatever he or she wants. Rights are always balanced with responsibilities by considering the broader interests of society at large. CCF's "personal choice" dogma creates the impression that the freedom to eat as one pleases (a right assumed to be on par with the freedom to speak or worship) is being trampled upon by those advocating for regulatory oversight of food corporations. But that's simply not so. The U.S. Constitution does not protect an individual's right to a Big Mac, or any other food. Also, even individual freedoms that are expressly guaranteed by the Constitution (such as free speech) are not absolute and are always balanced against the greater interests of society. (Whether *access* to truly nutritious food *should* be a basic human right guaranteed by the Constitution is another discussion altogether.)

> **When they say:** Big Brother is taking away your rights.
> **They assume:** Government is not already involved in our food choices.

When CCF sounds alarm bells about government on the march to do away with the American way of life and your freedom to enjoy your favorite foods, it conveniently glosses over the fact that government is already intimately involved in our food choices. Various federal agencies set standards for food safety, provide nutrition advice, subsidize agriculture, and otherwise oversee the types of foods we eat and the information we receive about them. Even "permissive policies," such as opening public school doors to soda companies, represent forms of government oversight. In fact, somewhere along the line, every food and beverage sold in the United States is already subject to some sort of government rule making. Food choices do not take place in a vacuum, but rather in the context of a domestic and global political economy driven by policies aimed at keeping the engine of capital operating smoothly. Many nutrition advocates are simply opposed to fueling that engine at the expense of public health; our objective, rather, is to work for government policies that are health-promoting and environmentally sustainable.

When they say: The food police are taking away your freedoms.

They assume: Nutrition advocates are targeting individuals.

The free-market doctrines promulgated by groups like CCF assume that the policy ideas of nutrition advocates pose an ominous threat to the freedoms and rights of consuming citizens. This is a clever inversion of nutrition advocates' objectives, which are not designed to usurp people's food choices, but rather to make healthier choices more available to everyone. In fact, the principal goal of shifting the emphasis away from individual behavior change is to establish government policies that hold corporations accountable, to foster an environment more conducive to making healthier food choices.

When they say: The food police think they know what's best for you.

They assume: Nutrition advocates want to punish people.

A key CCF ploy is to portray advocates of healthier eating as dour moralists who are overly invested in making people feel bad about their "wrong" food choices. Such grim scolds—the kind who know "what's best for you"—are likened to paternalistic nannies or, worse, oppressive Soviet-era tyrants bent on seizing your McFlurry with M&M's and replacing it with flavorless Party-issued alternatives. In the process, the final vestiges of rugged individualism are drained from the

American lifeblood. The truth is, most nutrition advocates don't want to punish anyone; nor do they wish to condemn people for their food choices. (There are notable exceptions, however, including some of PETA's campaigns, which in my opinion can be quite harsh and needlessly judgmental.) Rather, they seek government policies and corporate practices that make it easier for people to make healthier food choices.

Fighting Back: Exposing CCF's Hypocrisy

Another useful way to neutralize CCF's the-sky-is-falling hysteria about repressive food police is to expose its rampant hypocrisy. Fortunately, you'll find a veritable gold mine of material from the group itself. Here, then, are a few of CCF's duplicitous ideological bludgeons and some rejoinders.

Nutrition advocates have hidden or biased agendas

What could be more two-faced than an industry front group like the Center for Consumer Freedom accusing others of having "hidden agendas"? That this supposedly populist organization—which might be more accurately referred to as the Center for *Corporate* Freedom—has the gall to do so is mind-boggling and even amusing. The simplest way to respond to any argument made by CCF is to note that it is funded by the food, tobacco, and alcohol industries and represents their interests.

Wily food activists won't disclose their funding sources

Earlier, we saw how CCF likes to intimidate organizations like mine by demanding that they turn over financial records.

Yet while CCF is passionate about "exposing" advocacy groups' funding sources, it routinely refuses to open its own books to public scrutiny (more on this below). One would be hard-pressed to find a better illustration of a double standard.

We stand for consumer choice and democratic values

By opposing policies that would provide people with genuinely healthy food, CCF works to limit our food options to the processed products churned out by industry while keeping manufacturers firmly in control of the food discourse. It is the height of hypocrisy for CCF to espouse such ideals as freedom and democracy as it makes every effort to undermine our food choices. What's democratic about allowing a handful of multinational corporations to dictate what an entire nation—and indeed an entire planet—eats? If CCF were truly interested in freedom, it would let the democratic process unfold without interference from its strong-arm lobbying tactics. Indeed, if CCF really represents consumers, then why isn't it a membership organization? Where is the grassroots consumer movement banging on fearless leader Rick Berman's door begging for protection from the long arm of the food police? Where exactly are the consumers that the Center for Consumer Freedom purports to represent in the name of democracy?

Scare tactics? Radical activists? Them, not us!

We've seen many examples of the apparent relish that CCF takes in depicting nutrition advocates as despotic bogeymen bent on subverting the American way of eating. Such venom is just more of the pot calling the kettle black. Rather than cower before those working to safeguard public health, we should reserve our fear and trembling for CCF: its underhanded lobbying and scare tactics, its flat-out lies, its use of populist rhetoric to shill for corporate interests—the list of the group's disreputable maneuverings goes on.

CCF's efforts to portray sound nutrition policy reforms and those advocating for them as "radical" is likewise duplicitous. The truth is that CCF's corporate clients are the ones responsible for radicalizing the way Americans eat. In the blink of an evolutionary eye, we have gone from eating natural, nutrient-dense foods to factory-produced, highly processed, nutritionally deficient "products" that bear little resemblance to anything found in nature. Now that's radical.

Running Afoul of the Law?

In November 2004, Citizens for Responsibility and Ethics in Washington (CREW) filed a complaint with the Internal Revenue Service alleging that CCF violated its nonprofit, tax-exempt status. IRS law prohibits private individuals from benefiting from nonprofit organizations. But CREW alleges that director Rick Berman and his for-profit lobbying and public relations firm have received nearly $2 million from CCF and its predecessor organization since 1999. The Center for Media and Democracy notes that in the year 2000 alone, CCF paid $256,077 to Berman and Co., Inc. for "management services," although the organization did not report paying income to any of its employees.[14]

Tax-exempt organizations must have a charitable purpose. But according to CREW, CCF lobbies exclusively on behalf of food producers and the restaurant and tobacco industries and is "not remotely charitable."[15] Indeed, CREW notes that Rick Berman initially pitched the organization to Philip Morris as a vehicle to "unite the restaurant and hospitality industries in a campaign to defend against attacks from anti-smoking, anti-drinking, anti-meat activists." CREW's executive director, Melanie Sloan, said that, "Given all of the violations CCF has committed, a full and fair investigation should result in the organization losing its [tax] exemption."[16] (As of this writing, action on the complaint has yet to be taken.)

Who's Funding CCF? Who Can Tell?

Figuring out who, exactly, is funding CCF's operations is an ongoing challenge, considering that it—in classic front group style—works hard to keep that information secret. As a 501(c)(3) nonprofit organization, CCF is legally obligated to disclose certain financial information to the IRS and make it publicly available. CCF has complied with this requirement, but it has refused to reveal the identity of its funders. According to the Center for Media and Democracy, which inspected CCF's IRS filings for the year 2000, CCF declared a total income of $514,321, almost all of which came from seven unnamed donors.[17] Here is how CCF explains its secrecy regarding its funders:

> Many of the companies and individuals who support the center financially have indicated that they want anonymity as contributors. They are reasonably apprehensive about privacy and safety in light of the violence some activist groups have adopted as a "game plan" to impose their views.[18]

Bob Burton is editor of SourceWatch, an online project of the Center for Media and Democracy, which documents PR firms, front groups, and other organizations working to influence public opinion on behalf of corporations. His group has uncovered much previously undisclosed information about CCF's doings. (I highly recommend its Web site, SourceWatch.org, and sister site, PRWatch.org, as resources.) Burton says that CCF is using the threat of violence against its corporate funders as a "sham excuse" to hide their identities:

> Corporations sponsor front groups so that they can play ventriloquist to try and keep the gaze of journalists and the public fixed on the dummy. Of course CCF's sponsors demand secrecy; why else would they bother funding a front group? Secrecy is crucial to the success of both CCF and its corporate funders but doesn't play too well with the public. That's why CCF uses nonexistent violent threats to avoid disclosing the group's conflict of interest. Of course CCF knows this threat is a sham since director Rick Berman doesn't appear on television in disguise or use a pseudonym when talking to the media.[19]

Another curious thing about front groups like CCF is that food corporations can derive benefits from their slithery PR work without even paying for it. As Northeastern law professor Richard Daynard notes, the "smart folks" in the food business are happy to take advantage of the so-called free rider effect. They realize, explains Daynard, that "as long as CCF is doing it anyhow, why should a particular manufacturer pay for it, even if they like the service? The irony is that CCF is going to be funded by people who are behaving irrationally. If you're behaving rationally, you sit back and let other people fund them."[20]

FOOD ORGANIZATIONS CONTRIBUTING TO CCF (2001–2002)[21]

Applebee's International (restaurant chain—$15,000)

Dean Foods Company (dairy—$5,000)

Excel/Cargill (beef—$200,000)

Tyson Foods (chicken—$200,000)

Pilgrim's Pride (poultry—$100,000)

Perdue Farms (chicken—$40,000)

Coca-Cola Company ($200,000)

Outback Steakhouse (restaurant chain—$164,600)

Wendy's International ($200,000)

The Center for Media and Democracy obtained this information about corporate donations through an insider whistleblower.

Why It Matters

You might be thinking, so what? So what if Rick Berman and his cohorts want to run a few delirious Web sites and call some people names? What harm does it really do? Once you realize that CCF is funded by industry and serving its interests, isn't that enough to simply dismiss everything it does as the facile corporate toadying of another Washington lobby? Well, no, it's not that simple, because CCF is very effective at bringing its spin on food-policy issues to the media's—and hence the public's—regular attention. Indeed, we shouldn't underestimate its savvy use of the media to influence public opinion. (We will revisit CCF's tactics in later chapters.)

CCF's in-your-face smear tactics and other antics are tailor-made for a scandal-hungry press, which is always itching to entice readers and viewers with a good fight (staged or otherwise). CCF is thus well poised to position the food industry's worldview at the center of the "debate," whether or not conflict actually exists. Because "balance"-minded media outlets are perpetually anxious to present "both sides" of an issue, CCF's well-oiled PR machine is often able to step in and supply them with its own premanufactured controversy. So, for example, when a state proposes a school nutrition bill, CCF is on the spot, fulminating about how such policies are an egregious affront to students' "choices"—never mind the fact that such legislation typically enjoys overwhelming public support.

CCF speaks for a small segment of society—corporate elites—and its purpose is to portray those powerful minority interests as *universal* interests. This detail is rarely discussed in the mainstream media, which often can't even be bothered to disclose CCF's industry backing. (That fact is made clear on the "About Us" page of the group's Web site, but most reporters are apparently too uninterested, busy, or lazy to look it up.) Instead, the press presents CCF's line as simply another "side" of the discussion—and thereby sanctions its legitimacy and authority. That's why it's important to pay careful attention when CCF speaks.

When you have no interest in engaging in a serious, reasoned discussion of the issues but still want to defend yourself against your critics, your options are rather limited. You're basically left with distortions, lies, and emotionally exploitative vitriol as your rhetorical weapons. And that is CCF in a nutshell.

4

Nutriwashing Fast Food

There is no question that we make more money from selling hamburgers and cheeseburgers.[1]

—Matthew Paull, McDonald's chief financial officer

L et's be honest. McDonald's french fries taste good. Really good. Founder Ray Kroc didn't turn the fast-food chain into such a phenomenal success by selling lettuce. Good nutrition was about the last thing on the milkshake salesman's mind. Kroc's 1950s vision of dining has since spread to thirty thousand restaurants in 120 countries, serving fifty million customers a day and counting. That's a lot of burgers and fries. But this rapacious business model is not stopping McDonald's from trying to claim that it has the answer to America's health problems.

Years ago, the environmental movement coined the term "greenwashing" to describe how corporations use public relations to make themselves appear environmentally friendly. Today, nutrition advocates need their own moniker for a similar trend among major food companies—I like to call it "nutriwashing." As the food industry finds itself increasingly under attack for promoting unhealthy foods, one of its major defense strategies is to improve, or promise to improve, the nutritional content of its food.

Among the major peddlers of fast food, McDonald's has borne the burnt of the criticism from nutrition advocates, many of whom are especially troubled by the company's shameless marketing to children. In response, the corporation has developed a massive PR campaign aimed at convincing us that it really does care. But before believing the spin, we should ask whether these moves have any positive impact on the nation's health, or if, worse, the campaign could actually encourage people to eat more of the wrong foods.

Supersized Deceptions: Want McLies with That?

When it comes to putting our trust in a fast-food company, McDonald's gives us plenty of reasons to be skeptical. For example, in March 2004, just prior to the general release of the movie *Super Size Me* (which had already generated much publicity after winning the director's prize at the Sundance Film Festival), McDonald's made headlines by announcing its intention to stop supersizing fries and sodas. The company vehemently denied that its decision was in any way motivated by the film, in which director Morgan Spurlock documented the untoward effects of daily consumption of McDonald's fare on his own body, including near liver failure. Instead, the corporation insisted, the change was part of an overall plan to revamp its menu.[2] While the major media outlets were pre-dictably quick to celebrate the move, you only had to read the fine print to discover it was window dressing. The company merely eliminated its "supersize," 7-ounce french fries while maintaining the "large" 6-ounce portion, which is still signif-icantly bigger than the original 2.4-ounce portion that McDonald's began serving in the 1950s. Also, the available soda sizes would still range from 12 ounces to a whopping 32 ounces.

Moreover, although supersized soft drinks were removed as regular menu items, the products remain available as a "promotional option" for franchises. That explains why supersized drinks magically reappeared a little more than a year later in Chicago-area restaurants. During a one-month promotion, McDonald's customers who bought a Big Mac and fries could get a free 42-ounce beverage. For a Coke that means 410 calories and 28 teaspoons of sugar.[3] Nevertheless, McDonald's spokeswoman Anna Rozenich insisted, "This is not supersizing." She explained that franchises were being given flexibility to promote the humongous drinks "because competitors might be offering something like that" too.[4] So much for being a leader in responsible marketing; competition-driven fears over maintaining a healthy bottom line will trump concerns about the public's health every time.

Controversy over McDonald's misleading marketing tac-tics is nothing new. Indeed, various scams have embroiled the firm in prominent lawsuits in recent years. In one case, sev-eral vegetarian and Hindu groups charged the company with falsely claiming that its french fries were cooked in 100 percent vegetable oil, when they were in fact flavored with beef tallow.[5] The suit was eventually settled for $10 million and an apology. As of this writing, McDonald's is facing at least three more lawsuits accusing it of failing to disclose that its french fries contain potential allergens such as wheat and dairy. (The company maintains these ingredients are used simply as flavor enhancers.[6])

Another notorious case was filed in 2002 on behalf of two New York teens who ate regularly at McDonald's as children and are now suffering from diet-related health problems such as high cholesterol and diabetes. The plaintiffs allege the company deceptively promoted its food as nutritious. That case is still pending in federal court.

McDonald's 2002 promise to remove trans fat from its cooking oil in light of the substance being linked to increased heart disease also landed it in the courtroom. The original announcement garnered so much positive press that Stephen Joseph, the San Francisco lawyer who brought the case, called it the "most successful corporate PR campaign in history." Joseph estimates that 214 million people, or 70 percent of Americans, heard the news.[7] Although the company vowed to eliminate trans fat from its oil within six months, it failed to do so (claiming technical difficulties) and then made matters worse by not bothering to tell anyone. That's when Joseph decided to sue for fraud. McDonald's eventually settled the case in 2005 for $8.5 million.[8]

McDonald's trans fat troubles are far from over, however. As of this writing, not only has the company failed to fulfill its removal promise, but in February 2006, it "discovered" that its french fries actually contained a full one-third more trans fat than previously thought.[9] Considering that scientists say there is no acceptably safe level of trans fat for humans to consume, this is a significant discrepancy. Does this sound like a company we can trust to care about the public's health? What other McLies await unsuspecting consumers?

Maximizing the Halo Effect: McDonald's "Balanced Lifestyles"

By the time the obesity debate started heating up, McDonald's was already a company in need of serious spin control. So, in April 2004, with then U.S. secretary of Health and Human Services (HHS) Tommy Thompson at its side, McDonald's announced "an unprecedented, comprehensive balanced lifestyles platform to help address obesity in America and improve the nation's overall physical well-being."[10] Sounds very impressive, until you bother to scratch the surface. The major news outlets focused largely on the initiative's "Go Active! Adult Happy Meal" component, which included a "premium salad," bottled water, and a pedometer. Other "highlights" of the plan included how McDonald's promised to take an "industry-leading role" in working with HHS to determine the best way to "communicate" nutrition information to consumers. (Are the folks who invented the Big Mac really the best candidates for this job?)

An important concept in brand marketing is the "halo effect," which is the generalization of a positive feeling about a brand from one good trait.[11] In other words, if you think that a food company is selling healthy products, this can generate an overall good feeling about the company's brand. Whether or not the items are actually any healthier is beside the point.

Mary Dillon is responsible for McDonald's global marketing

strategy and brand development, as well as the company's Balanced, Active Lifestyles initiative. Here is how Dillon describes the effort: "McDonald's cares about the well-being of each of its guests throughout the world, and by making balanced, active lifestyles an integral part of the brand we aim to make a difference in this area of their lives."[12] In other words, McDonald's wants its customers to associate the *idea* of healthy lifestyles with its brand—a classic halo effect maneuver.

TIMING OF MCDONALD'S 2004 ANNOUNCEMENT

Announces phasing out of "super sizes" by year's end	March 2004
Announces "Balanced, Active Lifestyles Platform"	April 2004
General Release of *Super Size Me*	May 2004
Lawsuit filed against McDonald's over cooking oil	July 2004

A Salad in Name Only?

In 2003, the nonprofit Physicians Committee for Responsible Medicine (PCRM) conducted a nutritional analysis of thirty-four salads served at fast-food chains, and the results, to put it mildly, were dismal. The group awarded only two menu items (from Au Bon Pain and Subway) an "outstanding" rating for being high in fiber and low in saturated fat, cholesterol, sodium, and calories. McDonald's salads were among the worst offenders. PCRM noted that all of the corporation's salad entrées contain chicken (which has virtually as much cholesterol as beef) and concluded that the salads "may very well clog up your arteries." The group also awarded the

Bacon Ranch Salad with Crispy Chicken and Newman's Own Ranch Dressing "the dubious distinction of having the most fat of any salad rated. At 661 calories and 51 grams of fat, this salad is a diet disaster," with "more fat and calories and just as much cholesterol as a Big Mac."[13]

Curiously, when I checked the current data on the Bacon Ranch Salad with Crispy Chicken at the company's Web site, the numbers were different. (The salad is listed at 510 calories and 31 grams of fat.) When I asked dietitian Brie Turner-McGrievy (who conducted the PCRM study) to explain the discrepancy, she said that the site numbers must have changed, since she used data that was posted in 2003. She also noted that right after her group's study was released, McDonald's changed their nutrition facts to list all of the salads without chicken as an option. (This was not available prior to the survey.) "So we know they went back to look at their nutrition facts after our review. I wouldn't be surprised if they reanalyzed their salads—maybe using less dressing or less chicken—to come up with more favorable ratings," she said.[14]

Whatever the number of calories, merely calling something a salad doesn't make it healthy. Also, calling chicken "crispy" instead of fried is misleading. Essentially what McDonald's has done is taken the contents of its chicken sandwiches, dumped them on top of some lettuce, and served it up with a creamy dressing. As Bob Sandelman—whose market research firm specializes in the restaurant industry—told the press, food chains "have doctored those products up. If people really knew, they would find out that the salads pack more fat and calories. That's why the key word in all this is 'perceived' to be healthy."[15] The Fruit & Walnut Salad is better at 310 calories, but it's unlikely to hold you for a meal since it's just apples, grapes, and a few "candied walnuts," even with the "creamy low-fat yogurt."

McDonald's number-one motivation is to keep its customers addicted to its products, and lettuce covered with fried chicken furthers that goal. But touting its "premium salads" gives the false impression that the company sells healthy items.

California Cobb Salad (Grilled or Crispy Chicken)
Total Calories (with crispy and dressing): 490; fat: 27 g, sodium: 1,700 mg (71 percent of daily recommended)

Caesar Salad (Grilled or Crispy Chicken)
Total Calories (with crispy and dressing): 490; fat: 32 g; sodium: 1,520 mg

Bacon Ranch Salad (Grilled or Crispy Chicken)
Total Calories (with crispy and dressing): 510; fat: 31 g (almost half daily recommended); sodium: 1,670 mg (70 percent of daily recommended)

McSalad Deceptions[16]

Kids' Nutrition Also a Shell Game

In response to charges that it's turning a new generation of young people into loyal Big Mac and McFlurry fans, McDonald's now offers "Happy Meal Choices." The new and improved Happy Meal gives parents the option of replacing high-fat french fries with "Apple Dippers" (sliced apples and caramel dipping sauce). Instead of a Coke, kids can now have apple juice or milk. There is, however, no substitute for the hamburger, cheeseburger, or Chicken McNuggets.

But is this any real improvement? Probably not. For a toddler who needs about 1,000 calories per day, a Happy Meal consisting of four Chicken McNuggets, small french fries, and low-fat chocolate milk totals 580 calories, or more than half of a child's daily recommended calorie intake.[17] This of course says nothing about the dismal nutritional quality of these foods, which are devoid of fiber as well as vitamins and minerals that are especially important for growing children. And while it's true that the "Apple Dippers" in the Happy Meal contain fewer calories than french fries, this "improvement" hardly compensates for the heavy dose of sugar delivered by the dipping sauce that kids are sure to love.

Celebrity Halos and Target Marketing

Another time-honored marketing gimmick that McDonald's uses to maximum effect is celebrity endorsements. Back in 2003, the company had already entered into an exclusive marketing arrangement that cleverly linked Newman's Own "all-natural" salad dressings with McDonald's "premium" salad line. Newman's Own is a well-known name in the natural foods world, thanks largely to its founder, Paul Newman, who donates company profits to various charities. By hitching itself to Newman's star-powered and philanthropic wagon, McDonald's ensures extra-bonus halo effect. Never mind that the creamy dressings are dismally high in fat while the low-fat varieties are very high in salt. For example, a 1.5-ounce portion of Newman's Own Low Fat Balsamic Vinaigrette contains almost one-third of the day's recommended salt.[18] Natural does not always mean healthy.

Then, in 2005, McDonald's enlisted additional luminaries as pitch people for its new Fruit & Walnut Salad. The aim of this campaign was to associate the new salad with the celebrity cachet of young, healthy, thin, and hip superstars.

In announcing the effort, the company took the convenient opportunity to tie in its sponsorship of the world tour of pop music act Destiny's Child.[19] With tickets slated for sale just days later, McDonald's clearly had its sights set on the group's huge teenage audience, a demographic likely to be impressed by their musical icons' ostensible endorsement of the Fruit & Walnut Salad. That the Destiny's Child tie-in might also persuade young customers (and their friends) to order more "classic" varieties of junk food offers McDonald's a convenient side benefit that no doubt factored into the corporate PR strategy.

Another hip and healthy spokesperson jumping on the salad bandwagon was tennis champion Venus Williams. Dutifully issuing her own press release, she proclaimed, "As an athlete who is always on the go, I really appreciate the new Fruit & Walnut Salad. It is important to me that I can quickly grab a healthy nutritious meal on the run."[20] How many tennis matches (or even workouts) Williams can possibly sustain on 310 calories of apples and grapes is unclear, but what is certain is McDonald's determination to associate its brand with the vitality and success of one of the nation's most accomplished athletes.

Proving that no amount of positive PR is ever enough, another strategy tied to the new salad was the announcement of an "exclusive alliance" with nutritionist and author Dr. Rovenia Brock. Brock said she welcomed "the opportunity to collaborate with McDonald's to help spread the message of balance creation nationwide to key influencers and McDonald's customers nationwide—particularly African American families."[21] The precise meaning of "balance creation" and "key influencers" in this context is unclear at best. But along with coveting star endorsements from Destiny's Child and Venus Williams, this marketing tie-in is apparently part of McDonald's broader effort to include the African American community among its "key" marketing demographics.

Of course, targeting this audience was already an important business strategy for McDonald's, but with one notable difference: the type of food pitched. For example, in March 2005, just two months prior to the Fruit & Walnut Salad launch, McDonald's announced an offer to pay hip-hop artists in exchange for plugging Big Macs in their songs. Children's advocates and business observers alike were quick to condemn the move. "This campaign undermines McDonald's claim that they are serious about combating childhood obesity," said psychiatrist Alvin F. Poussaint, of the Judge Baker Children's Center and Harvard Medical School. Poussaint underscored hip-hop's enormous popularity with preteens and teens: "Even as McDonald's is drawing praise for pushing salads and apples, they are finding new ways to market high-calorie standbys like the Big Mac to children."[22] Similarly, *BusinessWeek* commentator David Kiley wrote:

> I happen to think McDonald's, for all the flack it gets about the childhood obesity problem, has a perfect right to sell Big Macs. But here's where the logic of this hip-hop plan jumps the rails for me. McDonald's just kicked off a campaign to advertise healthy eating and promoting physical activity to couch potato kids. Statistics are pretty clear that the obesity problem is especially bad among minorities in urban neighborhoods, arguably because there are more fast-food joints in

poor neighborhoods than produce stands and good-quality supermarkets.[23]

Journalist Sabrina Ford explains that the expropriation of hip-hop culture by the fast-food king is nothing new:

> McDonald's markets their chemically engineered goodies to black people using people who look like us and sound and act like they think we sound and act. What is so "premium" about a salad that includes fried, processed chicken? And I don't believe for one second that the members of Destiny's Child or the Williams sisters eat McDonald's on a regular basis. If you are going to use our culture as an attempt to speak to black people, please do so with respect.[24]

It's no surprise that McDonald's would want to play it both ways: while the company targets key markets with their standard fare by exploiting certain elements of pop culture (i.e., hip-hop), it also seeks to bask in the healthy glow exuded by other pop icons (i.e., tennis stars). In the end, everyone gets used and the only thing getting healthy is McDonald's profits.

It's the Burgers, Stupid: the Economics of Fast Food

It's really no wonder that McDonald's would have to rely on celebrity star power to sell the idea to the American public that its products are healthy. But it isn't some grand conspiracy theory that leads to me to believe that fast-food companies like McDonald's aren't actually providing healthier options. Rather, I simply observe the numerous signs that indicate that megachains are *incapable* of offering such fare, now or in the future. In the end, fast-food financial imperatives dictate what these companies can and cannot market. Let's take a closer look at this stark economic reality.

Small fraction of fast-food sales are healthier items

In 2005, McDonald's conceded that despite all the hoopla around its new salad offerings, only a tiny fraction of its customers actually orders them. While the company loudly trumpets the sale of 400 million premium salads since their introduction in 2003, that number is dwarfed by the total body count. McDonald's serves 23 million people a day in the United States alone, or roughly 16.8 billion people in the two-year period since the salads' introduction. As the *Washington Post* calculated, this means that in mid-2005 just 2.4 percent of McDonald's customers had ordered salads since they were added to the menu.[25]

We need look no further than the fast-food king itself to confirm these stats: McDonald's spokesperson Bill Whitman explained, "The most popular item on our menu continues to be the double cheeseburger, hands down."[26] McDonald's isn't alone in this regard. Data from NPD Foodworld indicate that the number-one entrée ordered by men in America is a hamburger and the number-one selection among women is french fries, followed by hamburgers.[27] Also, a typical Burger King outlet sells only 4 or 5 of its allegedly healthier Veggie Burgers in a day compared to 300 to 500 of any other sandwich or burger on the menu.[28]

Burgers are more profitable than salads

Fast-food chains are faced with unavoidable food-related obstacles when it comes to serving truly healthy alternatives. For example, produce is much harder to store than, say, frozen hamburger patties. Other challenges include standardization and mass production of messy, perishable fruits and vegetables. Such annoyances of nature add up to more complexity and higher costs. As Matthew Paull, McDonald's chief financial officer candidly explained to the *Economist* magazine, "There is no question that we make more money from selling hamburgers and cheeseburgers."[29]

As a result, one of the basic tenets of fast-food economics is the so-called 80-20 rule, which holds that 80 percent of a fast-food company's revenue derives from 20 percent of its products, usually its flagship line of burgers and fries. As *Forbes* magazine writer Tom Van Riper explains, so-called healthier fare at fast-food chains serves only a narrow fraction of the population while conveniently deflecting attention away from the remainder of the unwholesome menu:

> Certainly, soups and salads have added incremental revenue, since they serve that segment that has made a commitment to healthier eating. They also make for effective window dressing, helping to keep critics and regulators quiet. But a fast-food fixture that has measured its success in terms of "billions served" can't live on lightweight salads that people can get anywhere. It must beef up sales of Big Macs and Quarter Pounders. Given the 80-20 rule, a 5% drop in burger and fries sales, coupled with a 10% gain in

"new menu" items, would net out to a 2% drop in revenue. For a $20 billion company like McDonald's, that's a $400 million hit.[30]

McDonald's sales increases not due to salads (exactly)

Some media reports have attributed a recent upturn in McDonald's economic figures to the company's epiphany to sell so-called healthier fare. The funny thing is that McDonald's doesn't share this view. Bill Whitman, a company spokesperson, insists that the turnaround is actually due to wider and, in his view, "higher-quality" menu choices of all kinds, as well as cleaner stores.[31] (Founder Ray Kroc was obsessed with cleanliness.) Matthew Paull is more blunt. He freely admits that McDonald's sales growth is being driven by the "halo effect" visited upon the brand by the addition of (supposedly) healthier options, and he expects that trend to continue.[32]

People don't flock to fast-food chains for health food

Another sad economic truth is that most people simply do not choose to eat at a fast-food restaurant for the "health food" experience. Rather, price, convenience, and cleanliness are patrons' top priorities. According to one survey, only 4 percent cited availability of healthy food options as the most important reason for choosing a fast-food restaurant.[33] Part of the reason is that for most people, eating out represents a treat, while a healthy meal is something (in theory anyway) that people can make at home.

Who's eating the salads? Neutralizing the "veto vote"

An important marketing strategy is what's known in

restaurant lingo as "neutralizing the veto vote." This is when one member of a group (for example, a vegetarian) objects to the available menu choices, so the entire party goes elsewhere. Here's a typical scenario: a father and his children are hankering for burgers and milkshakes, but mom wants a salad. With a salad option on the menu, mom's veto vote is eliminated, and visiting McDonald's can once again be enjoyed by the entire family. In playing the salad card, McDonald's aim is therefore to lure not only the would-be naysayer back into its fold, but also the cash-carrying members of the veto voter's less fussy entourage—thereby positioning itself to sell *more* of its traditional unhealthy products. Indeed, *Forbes* magazine noted in 2004 that one of McDonald's "biggest coups has been getting mothers to order lunch while picking up Happy Meals for their kids. That rarely happened prior to the introduction of its salads in April 2003."[34] In another example of how McDonald's was aiming to fix a wasted customer opportunity, the *New York Times* reported that many parents "eat nothing while their children snack on burgers and fries."[35]

In other words, the people eating McDonald's salads are not current customers who are switching from eating burgers; rather, they are mostly people *who would otherwise not be McDonald's customers or would have ordered nothing*. This is important because I often hear nutrition advocates talk of "providing McDonald's customers with healthy alternatives," when the evidence strongly suggests that current customers aren't switching over, while new customers are just bringing others to buy more of the same crappy food. So where's the health benefit?

High cost of value meal marketing

Besides the element of speed, another main attraction of fast food is its low price. But patrons seeking to partake of McDonald's enlightened new product offerings will have to pony up handsomely for the privilege. The average price of a McDonald's salad, for example, is around four dollars—a full three dollars more than the classic items available on the "dollar menu," which include the double cheeseburger, the McChicken sandwich, fries, the assorted soft drink, and the hot fudge sundae. Also, at $5.99 a box, the (now defunct) Go Active! Adult Happy Meal was pretty steep compared to other (presumably less active) "meal combos."

A survey by the National Alliance for Nutrition and Activity (NANA) found that a McDonald's Quarter Pounder with cheese cost $1.41 less than a Quarter Pounder with cheese medium "extra value meal".[36] But who is going to let a measly $1.41 stand in the way of their stomach and an extra 660 calories? The NANA study also found that McDonald's did not offer "small" container sizes with such deals—so people whose principal motivation for eating at McDonald's is the low prices (meaning almost everyone) are effectively given an incentive to eat more food. Moreover, at most fast-food outlets these days it's hard to miss the dazzling "point of purchase" displays that encourage these combo meals.

When healthy doesn't sell, it's game over

Getting products (any products) into the mouths of cash-carrying customers is of course the top priority for food marketers. So when one of their creations fails to "show them the money," it gets swept into the dustbin of failed ideas. Such was the fate of the apparently less than popular Go Active! Adult Happy Meal, which was jettisoned by McDonald's after it had dutifully delivered the desired halo effect following the 2004 press conference. A nice McDonald's "customer satisfaction representative" apologized when I asked if it was still available, explaining that it was a "limited-time promotion."[37] Other "well-intentioned" menu innovations have also met their untimely demises at the hands of major restaurant chains. For example, in 2004 Ruby Tuesday reduced some portion sizes and added healthier items. However, when slumping sales threatened quarterly returns, the company soon returned to its roots, aggressively promoting its biggest burgers and restoring its larger portions of french fries and pasta. Similarly, while Wendy's garnered great press in February 2005 for its "bold" decision to add fresh fruit to its menu, that resolution was rescinded as soon as corporate headquarters reviewed the disappointing sales figures a few months later.[38] As the *Washington Post* explained in 2005, "Fast-food and casual dining chains are slowly going back to what they do best: indulging Americans' taste for high-calorie, high-fat fare."[39]

However warm and fuzzy the marketing may sound, the reality is that corporate sellers of fast food can only offer healthy options at the risk of going out of business. Nevertheless, health-themed campaigns such as McDonald's "premium salad" promotion are brilliant business strategies. Here's what fast-food giants get in return for investing some of their R&D and PR dollars in "healthier" products: (1) New business from veto voters and other "health-conscious" consumers; (2) business from veto voters' less health-minded friends and family members who will likely buy core (higher-profit-margin) products; (3) additional purchases from young people who, regardless of their interest in healthful eating, are lured in by endorsements by "cool" celebrities; (4) glowing press reports and overall great PR for undertaking a "bold" health initiative; (5) a reprieve from regulators and lawsuits, which are now deemed superfluous in light of new-found evidence of responsible corporate citizenship. With all of these corporate benefits, what do fast-food customers gain? Just a lot of spin.

Why We Can't Expect McDonald's to Make "Healthy Food"

One of my biggest frustrations is hearing nutrition advocates say things like, "We should applaud McDonald's for adding healthy menu items," or that offering any salads is "a step in the right direction." While I certainly sympathize with the view that fast-food chains should provide healthy options, several aspects of this way of thinking just don't sit well with me.

For one, this position encourages and reinforces self-regulation as a viable model for social change. But as we have seen, voluntary measures are subject to the whims of quarterly profit earnings. Too often, Big Food's promises don't last longer than the time it takes for the ink to dry on a corporate press release. It simply goes against the basic tenets of market economics to ask corporations to put public interest ahead of profits. It's not McDonald's job to promote public health under our economic system. What *is* McDonald's job is to expand market share and maximize profits for shareholders, period. Expecting a corporation to voluntarily behave in a way that is antithetical to its mandate is a hope-less cause. (The only variation on this rule is when a company is financially threatened, such as by litigation or regulation, in which case the move is not truly voluntary. And even then, the policy change is an economic risk/benefit calculation.)

Advocates who choose to applaud companies like McDonald's for taking steps "in the right direction" or for trying to be "part of the solution" shouldn't be surprised to feel frustration and disappointment when companies renege—as they invariably do—on their "well-intentioned" pledges. I also fear the loss of credibility that comes when public health advocates show appreciation for ultimately short-lived corporate policy changes. Why exactly do corpo-rations deserve any credit for slightly scaling back on their overall abysmal behavior? It's just not our job as health advo-cates to applaud corporate behavior, no matter how "favor-able" the move might appear. Companies have well-paid PR departments to pat themselves on the back ad nauseum. When health leaders add to that positive spin, it just plays right into the hands of corporations by allowing them to essentially co-opt the national dialogue around nutrition policy and encourages them to roll out more meaningless "initiatives."

But in the end, it's simply not economically feasible for fast-food companies to serve truly healthy fare, because they can make more money selling high-fat, high-sugar, and high-fat products. That's why the chains have every incentive to showcase their best-selling, highest-profit-earning items, while relegating allegedly healthier alternatives to the safer, positive-PR-generating periphery.

But, I hear my colleagues object, the "reality" is that people will continue to eat at fast-food chains, so we must accept that and convince companies like McDonald's to provide better choices. But why must we resign ourselves to a model that corporate America has created for us? Is a little tinkering around the edges really the best we can hope for? Moreover, in confining their complaints against fast food to a narrow set of health-related issues (e.g., portion sizes), advocates ignore a host of other critical social ills for which many food corporations are also responsible—including unjust labor practices, environmental destruction, cruelty to animals, and so forth.[40] One of my biggest frustrations with many nutrition advocates is their unwillingness to address this much bigger (and ultimately more important) picture.

Indeed, if nutrition advocates limit their agendas to extracting minor concessions from large companies—such as the addition of salad—we are unlikely to even get to ask larger questions about what's wrong with the entire food system. Of course, this narrowly defined model of corporate behavior change suits Big Food just fine because it keeps them in the driver's seat and doesn't threaten their overall business model or very existence. (In contrast, an entire movement of activists is working hard to create sustainable, healthy, and just alternatives to the current corporate food system model; more on this later.)

The question, therefore, should not be, "How can McDonald's play a positive role in promoting public health?" but rather, "What economic and political forces have allowed the fast-food industry to change, virtually overnight, the human diet that nature provided us throughout evolution?"

The question is not how we can tweak the business practices of a few major corporate players, but rather how we can remove the current system from our path so that we can make way for a better alternative? How can we create truly healthy alternatives that resemble how humans are meant to eat, instead of how corporations would have us eat?

We cannot rely on the same industry that is partly responsible for getting us into this mess to get us out of it. Instead, we need to look for better answers. But first, we need to stop allowing the likes of McDonald's to define the questions.

Ten Tips for Reading a Fast-Food Press Release

1. Always look at what exactly the company is promising to do. Often the rhetoric sounds better than the reality. Be wary of secondhand media accounts and always read the original press release.
2. Note the timing of the announcement. Is the company trying to fend off negative criticism related to a recently released report, book, or film?
3. See who is making the announcement. Remain skeptical of celebrity endorsements, especially with cross-promotions (such as concerts).
4. If a company is promoting a new healthy menu item, the first question should be, how does it stack up against more traditional offerings nutritionally? For example, are there any nutritional advantages to a "salad" that essentially consists of sandwich ingredients in a bowl? Also, creamy dressings can cause salads to top burgers in calories.
5. Look out for euphemisms such as "crispy" and

"batter-dipped"—which are usually corporate-speak for "deep-fried."

6. See how much more expensive the new "healthier" item is than the core products. Is the company offering the new healthier option as part of any or their usual "value meals"? If not, this lowers incentives for purchase.

7. Notice any timetable for the company's promised reform. A common trick is to set the actual date of implementation far in the future, or use vague language. Key words to watch for include *phasing* and *testing*. McDonald's, for example, announced in March 2004 its intention to "phase out" supersizing by the end of that year, a full nine months out.

8. Look for loopholes and exceptions that function as end runs around supposed policy reforms—e.g., McDonald's decision to allow supersizing "for promotions."

9. See if the company has followed through on its promises. If it hasn't, use that as evidence of how they can't be trusted.

10. Look out for reversals in policy or "limited-time offers." These are often hard to spot, since companies don't usually announce them. For example, McDonald's introduced its Go Active! Adult Happy Meal with much fanfare, but conveniently said nothing about the item being a limited promotion.

5

Nutriwashing
Processed Foods

The food industry is in a better position to educate consumers than anyone else.[1]

—Cal Dooley, Food Products Association

You could easily be thinking, as you walk down the supermarket aisle, that the snack sections have been transformed into an oasis of whole-grain natural potato chips, granola bars, and wheat-berry juice. Have you tried those Whole Grain Chips Ahoy cookies? They are good for you now. Did you realize that Cheetos Jumbo Puffs Flamin' Hot Cheese Flavored Snacks are trans fat free? Aren't you relieved that your children are now drinking soft drinks that provide them proper hydration?

That's how the big food corporations want you to feel as they bathe their products in the warm, fuzzy glow of health-themed marketing and PR. I also call their efforts "nutriwashing."

Mounting awareness that out-of-control junk food consumption may have something to do with obesity and other diet-related public health problems has sent shivers down the spines of corporate food makers. Up until a few years ago, the products of industry giants like Kraft Foods, Frito-Lay, and General Mills—fixtures in household cupboards and lunch pails across the nation—enjoyed relatively squeaky-clean reputations. Setting their PR machines into overdrive, the few large firms dominating today's increasingly consolidated food market are attempting to burnish their corporate images and protect their bottom lines against the nagging perception that something is amiss. While fast-food chains like McDonald's face formidable obstacles when it comes to playing the "health" card, packaged-food companies are quickly discovering many clever to ways to position themselves as "part of the solution."

Reformulating Whole Grains into Half-truths

Let's be honest about what makes the major packaged-food companies so successful: they process the hell out of food. As mentioned previously, industrial food manufacturing involves appropriating raw materials from nature and turning them into profitable commodities. That perfectly describes what happens when Kellogg takes whole corn, strips it of almost all naturally occurring nutrients, adds sugar, salt, and chemical additives to maximize flavor, stability, and shelf life, and puts the ingredients through a complex manufacturing process. Out pop Corn Pops. A similar fate has befallen pretty much every flour-based product on supermarket shelves: cereals, breads, crackers, chips, cookies, cakes, and so on—all major sources of excess calories and a serious threat to America's health.

In contrast, whole, unprocessed grains are rich in fiber and nutrients, and can contribute significantly to good health. Their regular consumption is associated with a decreased risk of heart disease and certain cancers, for example. That's why the federal government's updated 2005 Dietary Guidelines for Americans urges people to increase their daily intake of whole grains.[2] In fact, the guidelines offer a long overdue explanation for why it is important from a nutritional standpoint to choose whole-grain foods such as brown rice over products made with highly processed white flour. (This recommendation is an important rebuff to the recent "low-carb" craze, which needlessly made many Americans fearful of healthful complex carbohydrates.)

While federal nutrition guidelines are never as clear as they should be, the government's advice is essentially to eat more grains in their natural, unprocessed form, rather than those that come in relatively nutrient-deficient packaged products. But food manufacturers—never willing to let nutrition details stand in the way of a good marketing opportunity—have appropriated this recommendation for their own purposes. Now, the dietary guidelines are simply a tool for marketing reformulated "whole grain" versions of "classic" junk foods—products that remain nutritionally deficient despite the nominal addition of whole grains. Indeed, look high and low through the dietary guidelines and you'll be hard-pressed to find a recommendation for anything resembling Whole Grain Reese's Puffs, Whole Grain Chips Ahoy, or Whole Grain Wonder Bread.

General Mills Cereals: the Whole Grain Chutzpah Award

General Mills is a top seller of children's cereals, with annual sales of more than $1 billion. On the heels of the dietary guidelines update in January 2005, the company announced (with much fanfare) the launch of reformulated "whole grain" versions of its cereals. To ensure maximum "point-of-purchase" visibility, the boxes were plastered with huge

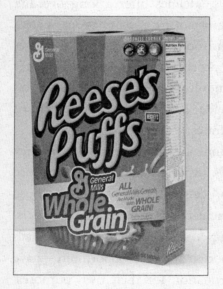

"whole grain" banners. And in April 2005, when the government released a revamped food pyramid— the graphic that illustrates the principles of the guidelines—General Mills was also quick to place the new image (called MyPyramid) on its cereal boxes. The corporation's self-congratulatory take on its product makeovers was clear at a 2005 Federal Trade Commission meeting on food marketing and childhood obesity. Here Kendall Powell, a General Mills vice president, spoke glowingly of the nutritional advantages afforded by the revamped products: "Obesity," he said, "is about calories and cereal is a low-calorie way to start the day."[3] Of course good nutrition isn't only about calories; it's also about the actual nutrients (or lack thereof) in the food.

Apparently, no cereal is too absurd for General Mills to label "whole grain." Conspicuously absent from Powell's dog and pony show were mentions of General Mills cereals aimed at children, such as Whole Grain Reese's Puffs, Whole Grain Cookie Crisps, Whole Grain Cocoa Puffs, Whole Grain Lucky Charms, and Whole Grain Chocolate Lucky Charms. And no wonder, given that Lucky Charms, for instance, is composed of whole-grain oats, sugar, canola oil, and marshmallows, which are made up of sugar, corn starch, corn syrup, dextrose, gelatin, two yellow dyes, blue dye, red dye, and artificial flavor. But just in case you, concerned parent, were beginning to suspect that "nutrition" is not actually lurking somewhere in this bewildering morass of ingredients, a "whole grain" banner is draped prominently across the Lucky Charms box for your edification and convenience.

How then does General Mills explain this "sugary whole grain" contradiction? The company argues that high sugar content is basically unimportant, given the products' overall nutritional benefits. Here's how Marybeth Thorsgaard, a General Mills spokesperson, justified it to me: "Even with presweetened cereals, there really is no better breakfast your child could eat in the morning. Presweetened cereals account for less than 5 percent of your sugar for the entire day, but because it's fortified and nutritionally dense for the amount of calories, there really is no better breakfast that your child could eat."[4] Using the passive voice in conjunction with the corporate-speak term "presweetened" makes it sound as if the added sugar occurs *naturally*. And no better breakfast? Compared to what? Starving? Marion Nestle, nutrition professor at New York University and author of *Food Politics*, is unconvinced: "It's hard not to react sarcastically to such statements from cereal makers. I have heard them say the reason sugary cereals are good for kids is because of the milk that's added. That, I suppose, would also be the rationale for giving kids cookies for breakfast. This is a marketing ploy to make people think that whole grain Cocoa Puffs are healthy. Sugar is still the first ingredient."[5]

Dietitian Fern Gale Estrow is also skeptical about the General Mills reformulation scam and is concerned that parents might be duped by the new labels:

> The level of confusion in nutrition is already massive. Now we have whole grain Lucky Charms. I think it's totally bogus. The dietary guidelines were changed to make a stronger statement about fiber, and this product has less than one gram of fiber per serving. That's just not sufficient. The company is entitled to reformulate its products, but please don't market them as whole grain, because that is not the issue. Is it an improvement, yes, is it an improvement that warrants the level of celebration they are giving it, no. It's a brilliant marketing strategy, if you think about it, given the amount of free press they are getting.[6]

Reformulating products with whole grain is just one recent addition to the processed-food industry's burgeoning bag of marketing tricks. Touting products as "zero trans fat" is another popular promotion ploy, especially since the feds added trans fat to the required "Nutrition Facts" label. Regardless of whether they ever contained the artery-congesting substance to begin with, many otherwise nutritionally dismal items now sport trans fat free labels like badges of honor. Among my favorite examples is Frito-Lay's "zero trans fat" Chicago Steakhouse Loaded Baked Potato Flavored Potato Chips. (I don't know what "steakhouse loaded" means and I am not sure I want to.) Containing or not containing one particular ingredient does not a health food make.

Controlled Portions of Junk Food: Paying More to Get Less

In addition to the poor nutritional content of most processed food, another problem health advocates complain about is how portion sizes have ballooned in recent years, distorting Americans' perception of what constitutes a normal serving. Without missing a beat, food companies have rushed to the rescue with their own techno-fix solutions to this, too. In 2003, Kraft Foods (which owns Nabisco brands) vowed to reduce portion sizes in the name of public health. But less than a year later, the company had a change of heart and decided instead to give consumers the option of purchasing snacks that are predivided into "100-calorie packs"—whose ostensible purpose is to deter consumption of the entire box in a single sitting. (As if tearing open consecutive packages wouldn't occur to anyone.) Kraft has magnanimously offered to save consumers from themselves by marketing overly packaged, environmentally destructive, and (most significantly) higher-priced portion-control versions of Chips Ahoy cookies and Cheese Nips, among other favorites.

Also jumping on the preportioning bandwagon is General Mills, who has divided some of its Pop-Secret microwave popcorn bags into 100-calorie segments, while Procter & Gamble now sells canisters of Pringles brand potato chips that are split into 100-calorie single-serve polypropylene cups. Marketing expert John Stanton explains that because the "portionability" maneuver allows corporations to charge a premium for the product, it's a clear "win for the business," even though Stanton cautions food sellers that their packages "better make it clear why you're paying more to get less."[7] Of course, eating less processed food is better. Just don't let it fool you into thinking you're eating healthfully. One hundred calories of junk food is still junk.

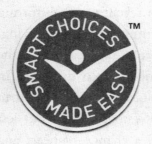
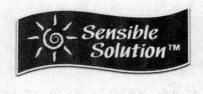

Smart and Sensible: Sealing the Deal with Spotty Solutions

In addition to recent marketing developments, many traditional nutriwashing tactics remain quite popular. For example, food companies have been adorning product labels with boastful health claims for years. While the "Nutrition Facts" label that appears on the back or the side of a package is heavily regulated by the federal government, it's pretty much a free-for-all when it comes to the front, where you'll often find eye-catching "callouts" such as "fat free" and "all natural." With few standards (government or otherwise) to define the meaning of such claims, corporations are liberally enlisting them to get you, gullible consumer, to fall for them at the most critical and influential location—store shelves.

To hear food companies tell it, such marketing tactics are innocently designed to "educate" consumers, providing them with crucial information that neither advocacy groups nor ill-funded government oversight agencies are able to convey. So where else can consumers find the information they seek but from the food makers themselves? As the *Washington Post* sadly noted in 2005, "Product packaging is the second most common place where people get their nutrition advice, after their doctors."[8] But is this a good idea? While the Food and Drug Administration has established rules (albeit poorly enforced ones) for the specific types of "health claims" that a food company can make, some manufacturers are essentially doing an end run around these directives with their own "seal programs." Now, two of the largest food companies, PepsiCo and Kraft, are awarding their own self-congratulatory stamps of approval to their products. For consumers, the result can only be more confusion. Here is how dietitian and columnist Melinda Hemmelgarn explains what's going on:

> If you're a food company, having a health claim on your product label makes good business sense. But what if your food product doesn't meet the stringent requirements of the FDA's health claims? One option would be to establish your own in-house system and affix a unique symbol on your company's food packages, setting those products you deem "healthier" apart

from others. That's exactly what PepsiCo and Kraft have done.[9]

Indeed, PepsiCo has developed a "Smart Spot" graphic to signify its "healthier" alternatives, while Kraft has stamped its supposedly more wholesome offerings with a "Sensible Solutions" icon. Both companies use green as the main color in their seal logos, since everyone knows that green means "healthy," not to mention "go." With the Smart Spot, PepsiCo is plainly telling you that it's smart to choose these products, and who doesn't want to be smart? The check mark symbol is also designed to make people's lives simpler—as summed up neatly in the Smart Spot tagline, "Smart Choices Made Easy." When PepsiCo launched the program in early 2005, it described the Smart Spot "as a shortcut, an easy way for consumers to identify a broad range of food and beverage choices from PepsiCo that contribute to a healthier lifestyle."[10] Similarly, Kraft encourages consumers to be sensible and choose products with its own version of a green seal. Of course, it wouldn't be either smart or sensible to, say, not buy these companies' products at all. Or would it?

Through the Eyes of the Brands

When most people hear "Pepsi" they think of the soda. But unlike Coca-Cola, which is exclusively a beverage maker, PepsiCo manufactures food products, too—a lot of them. In fact, thanks to market consolidation, the corporation has become one of the world's largest food and beverage companies, with 2005 revenues of more than $32 billion.[11] Familiar brand names under PepsiCo's control include Frito-Lay, Gatorade, Tropicana, and Quaker Oats. Snack-food giant Frito-Lay, which makes up one-third of PepsiCo's total sales, is, as one business analyst put it, "the undisputed chip champ of North America."[12] Lay's potato chips, Doritos, Tostitos tortilla chips, and Cheetos snacks *each* generate more than a staggering $1 billion in annual sales.[13]

Clearly, PepsiCo is a company with a lot of salty snacks on its hands. So the task of reinventing itself as a health-promoting, responsible corporate citizen in a highly competitive market is a formidable challenge to say the least. Despite reports that only 10 percent of survey participants rated the food giant as being "concerned with my health," placing it near the bottom of corporate rankings,[14] PepsiCo remains adamant about positioning itself as "part of the solution."

PepsiCo made its case loud and clear at a January 2005 workshop in which the Institute of Medicine (IOM), a government advisory agency, was considering untoward effects of junk food marketing on children. All the major food companies were represented, each falling over the other in an effort to prove how bound and determined it was to address the problem. Ellen Taaffe, PepsiCo's vice president of "Health and Wellness Marketing," explained how marketing experts had advised her firm that "we were a different company than most and we needed to get the story out."[15] By this she meant that PepsiCo had a diverse array of products that could be positioned as healthy, if only done the right way. "So we thought about it and we realized that we really have a consumer story here. And we have a way to help moms make some healthier choices to help move their families toward healthier lifestyles; and thus the creation of the Smart Spot program."[16] (This patronizing use of the term *moms* is quite popular among food-industry spokesmen and spokeswomen alike; apparently, for these executives, "dads" don't do any shopping or care about their children's health; and with all the time pressure that working mothers face these days, companies are happy to exploit this with fancy-labeled convenience foods.)

At the IOM workshop, Taaffe further explained that after conducting about twenty focus groups, PepsiCo found that the Smart Spot seal was "a big help to moms":

> It helps cut through the clutter, once they understand the program, it helps them to make choices, in ways that are familiar to them and with brands that they love and great-tasting products. They wanted the credit for making smart choices. That was the way they could feel good about making little steps and those little steps combined can really make a big difference in their families' lives. We started advertising this through the eyes of the brands, which is how consumers know us. Consumers don't know us, or probably don't care that it's PepsiCo, but they know the brands and what that brand means in their life.[17]

You probably have to be a food-company executive to understand exactly how brands have eyes, and how to advertise through them. But what Taaffe is essentially saying is that the company's brand images are what sell the products, and that this is the focus of the Smart Spot campaign. As an example, she showed IOM committee members an ad for Quaker oat-meal and quoted from the copy: "It's the delicious way to help lower cholesterol; it's the family tradition that helps warm you all over. It's the Smart Spot, the symbol of smart choices made easy. Find it on Quaker oatmeal, proven to help lower cholesterol after just 30 days as part of a healthy diet, one of over 100 smart choices from PepsiCo." The family tradition that warms you all over plus lowers cholesterol: now what could be smarter than that?

Getting the Lingo Down: The Good, the Better, and the Ugly

Of course, PepsiCo hasn't gotten rid of all the products that don't meet its own self-selected criteria for the Smart Spot seal. From a marketing perspective, this puts the company in a bit of a bind: how to position the new products as healthy without giving consumers the impression that the old products are, well, unhealthy, or even worse, unworthy of purchase. No worries—PepsiCo pitch people found a clever way around this temporary impasse. They just created a new language for talking about the products, a new classification scheme aimed at showcasing each item in its best light. PepsiCo has divided its products into "good for you" and "better for you" (the Smart Spot offerings), and "product alternatives" and "fun-for-you" foods (non–Smart Spot items). Confused? Maybe PepsiCo vice president Ellen Taaffe can help clarify the distinction:

When we say "good-for-you" products, these are products that are actively good for you, such as Quaker Oats, Tropicana, Aquafina water. And when we say "better-for-you," we mean products that are better than a product alternative, so products that are reduced in sugar or fat, like a product like a Diet Pepsi or a product like Baked Lays. We also make some functional products that are actively good for you, products like Gatorade, which has been proven to hydrate athletes better than water. That part of our portfolio is 30 percent and that surprises a lot of people.[18]

What I find most disturbing about this corporate-speak is how PepsiCo gets to be the authority on defining what "healthy" means, while conveniently using as the basis for comparison the company's least-healthy products. Of course, if you start with crap, anything slightly less crappy can be defined as "better-for-you." (Just like, compared to starving, Reese's Puffs cereal could be a better option.)

Adrift in the Nutriwash

As of 2005, more than two hundred products—including Gatorade, Diet Pepsi, and Baked Lay's—sported the Smart Spot symbol. But simply labeling a product healthy doesn't make it so. Chips are still full of salt and chemical additives, and have a nutritional profile on a par with diet sodas, which are completely devoid of nutrients and contain artificial sweeteners and other potential health hazards.

PepsiCo earns its place next to General Mills for the chutzpah award in finding no cereal too sugary to call healthy. Among the kid-friendly breakfast cereals deemed worthy of basking in the healthy glow of the Smart Spot are Peanut Butter Crunch, Cap'n Crunch Swirled Berries, and

Cap'n Crunch MagiColor Berries. How exactly is Cap'n Crunch Swirled Berries construed as "better for you"? According to Team Smart Spot, it's because the product is made with one-third less sugar than its "original" counterpart. Leave it to corporate America to put a ton of sugar in a product and then turn around and tout a modest cutback in the ingredient as a health benefit.

The low-sugar cereal scam prompted a California woman to file a lawsuit under the state's consumer protection laws against Kraft, General Mills, and Kellogg in 2005. She alleges that the companies' low-sugar cereals falsely represent "that they offer a nutritional advantage over defendants' full-sugar breakfast cereal products, when in fact, the removed sugar is replaced by other carbohydrates, thus offering no significant nutritional advantage."[19] Just a few months later, a similar case was filed in Montreal against Kellogg Canada.[20]

Nutrition consultant Fern Gale Estrow is especially troubled about the psychological impact of Smart Spot marketing on children. Kids, says Estrow, are easily manipulated by the cross-culturally recognizable, green=go symbol and its approving check mark: "A check mark means something is OK, no matter what language you speak."[21] What better way to get kids to identify a product as good and healthy than by putting a happy-looking check mark on the packaging?

Wellness as a Growth Opportunity: Keeping Profits Healthy

One of the ways that food corporations legitimate their slick nutriwashing campaigns is by pitching them as great business "opportunities" that are a win-win for consumers and their bottom lines alike. PepsiCo executives, for example, love to talk about the how the Smart Spot program is poised to tap into the burgeoning "health and wellness" market—a "growth driver," in industry-speak—thus positioning the firm to "do well by doing good." As company vice president Ellen Taaffe insists, "Wellness will be one of the growth trends over the next several decades. If we can develop better-tasting, convenient, and healthier fare, we have hit gold."[22] In fact, the company claims that revenue growth for Smart Spot products is twice that of its "fun-for-you" products,[23] giving the impression that PepsiCo is being rewarded with positive financial results. On closer inspection, however, this claim is yet another example of corporate spin: by definition, any *new* category of products will have more "growth" potential than an existing category simply because it's starting from scratch; unlike established brands, many of which have been around for decades, the new nutri-washed products simply have more room to "grow." Why is this important? Because it's disingenuous for PepsiCo to claim it will be forever more motivated to promote so-called healthier products based on misleading early growth claims.

The best way to find out the truth about the real motivations behind nutriwashing efforts like PepsiCo's Smart Spot program is to read the business press. When the audience is other businesspeople, food-company executives are more likely to be honest and up-front than they are with journalists from general-audience publications (or certainly at government hearings on health policy). Thus, when asked by *Smart-Money* magazine about how "the new focus on health by consumers" was changing business, PepsiCo CEO Steve Reinemund was surprisingly blunt:

As it happens right now, our healthy alternatives—we call them our Smart Spot alternatives—are growing at a faster rate because that's where consumers are moving. But over time I believe that equilibrium between health and wellness and indulgence is really where the consumer will be.[24]

Reinemund essentially admits that the current growth of PepsiCo's new "health and wellness" category is a temporary phenomenon. Sales of these products, he concedes, will eventually even out to a level similar to that of the company's more established "indulgence"—i.e., unhealthy—brands. Either way, it's win-win for PepsiCo. While the public is hoodwinked into thinking that the company is making healthier products, sales in all categories continue unabated. But what doesn't change is Americans' poor health.

Kraft's Crafty Nutrition Criteria

Hoping to avoid embroiling itself in the kinds of litigation and PR nightmares that plagued its tobacco-selling sister company Philip Morris, Kraft Foods has positioned itself alongside PepsiCo and other top food sellers as "part of the solution" to obesity. In 2003, Kraft announced its intention to devote a major portion of its $350 million-plus research and development budget to the creation of myriad "healthier" product options. In a two-year period, the food maker reformulated some 750 items, or more than 10 percent of its total sales by volume. "This is the single largest reformulation effort ever undertaken by the company," said Lance Friedmann, Kraft's senior vice president for global health and wellness.[25] The company promised, moreover, that by the end of 2005, 25 percent of its products would "qualify" for its Sensible Solutions flag.[26]

But can a company that built its fame and fortune on Oreos, Cheez Whiz, and Cool Whip really reformulate its way out of a public health crisis? I asked Dr. Renu Mansukhani, health policy consultant with the advocacy group Parents' Action for Children, to evaluate the nutrition criteria of both the PepsiCo Smart Spot and the Kraft Sensible Solutions initiatives. She noted that both companies claim their nutrition standards are based on "government statements." While PepsiCo has at least made an effort to identify those statements, Mansukhani said it's unclear (at least from the corporation's Web site) exactly what government guidelines Kraft is using in its Sensible Solutions program.

Furthermore, while PepsiCo uses the same set of nutrition criteria to assess products within each of three product categories (beverages, meals, and snacks), Kraft employs a different set of nutrition standards for almost every type of food—a strategy that Mansukhani calls "sneaky."[27] Also, if an item in the "cookies and crackers" category doesn't meet the first or second set of nutrition criteria that Kraft has established for it, it can still earn the Sensible Solutions approval stamp if one of two additional criteria are met; according to Kraft, the product "must be free of or low in calories, fat, saturated fat, sugar, or sodium, or must have 25 percent less of one of these in comparison to the base product or an appropriate reference product; and must be reviewed by Nutrition Department."[28] (Confused? Me, too, but don't you feel better knowing that Kraft's Nutrition Department is on the job?) It seems that getting a product like Chips

Ahoy cookies to qualify for a Sensible Solutions seal is a formidable task, so Kraft decided to help things along by giving (for example) CarbWell Chips Ahoy a free pass as long as the sugar content is 25 percent lower; but if not, comparing it to some other product will also suffice—you know, whatever works.

Mansukhani's main concern is that programs like Sensible Solutions are seducing people into purchasing products falsely marketed as "healthy." "We know it's happening," she says. "People are doing the best they can, buying these products thinking they will help them eat better, but that's not necessarily true."[29] Mansukhani also worries that such campaigns could even cause people to eat more unhealthy food— a phenomenon known as the "SnackWell effect," named after the famed brand of low-fat cookie that some people eat more of in the mistaken belief that low in fat also means low in calories. Perhaps not coincidentally, the SnackWell product line is owned by Kraft Foods.

The Hidden Dehydration Epidemic

While nutrition advocates are busy sounding alarm bells about diet-related threats to health such as obesity and diabetes, the marketers of "sports drinks" are trying to convince us that we (especially children) are imperiled by another malady altogether: severe dehydration. PepsiCo's Gatorade—a product that has achieved near-cult status in many school athletic programs— backs up its claims about the superior hydrating capacities of the product based on "findings" of the impressive-sounding Gatorade Sports Science Institute (which is of course funded by the company itself). Any nutritionist not on a corporate payroll will tell you that Gatorade's hydration claims are essentially bogus. Dietitian Melinda Hemmelgarn, for example, notes that "Gatorade is simply sugar and water; it's not a healthy product."[30] Moreover, Dr. David Ludwig, director of the obesity program at Children's Hospital Boston, says that most studies showing a hydration benefit with sports drinks apply only to triathletes. Ludwig stressed that "kids are not triathletes" and that sports drinks would come in handy only if dehydration were suddenly to become a public health menace.[31]

Likewise troubled by the burgeoning "thirst epidemic," Coca-Cola has positioned its Powerade line of "high-performance" beverages—some of which ironically contain high levels of caffeine—to respond to the problem. A Powerade product called Advance, for instance, is marketed as combining "the energy you want with the hydration you need."[32] The Advance campaign is part of a broader advertising push by Coke, launched in February 2006, to drive home the message that "[a]ll beverages, including those that contain caffeine, contribute to proper hydration,"[33] which is like saying, "All foods, including those that don't, contribute to a healthy diet." (Oh wait, food companies say that, too.) That caffeine is a diuretic and a known cause of excessive urination and dehydration is a fact conveniently ignored.[34]

Another popular "dehydration-relief" product is Kraft's Capri-Sun Sport drink, an item that is marketed heavily to children. While the drink has more sugar and calories than the company's other Sensible Solutions beverages, it still qualifies for the seal of approval. Why? Because Kraft claims (right on the front of the box) that the drink "hydrates better than water." According to the *Wall Street Journal*,[35] Kraft funded a study of twenty-nine children between the ages of nine and twelve. The children exercised and on breaks were allowed to take a drink. On average, the kids drank more Capri-Sun Sport than water. I tried to track down the actual study results (which, as it turns out, have not yet

been published in a peer-reviewed journal) to see if that was really how Kraft determined its drink had a nutritional benefit—simply because kids drank more Capri-Sun than water. I learned that the

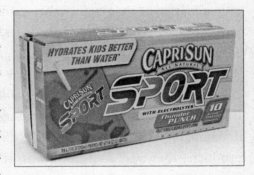

kids were placed on exercise equipment for eighty-minute sessions in hot and humid weather[36] (this is how most "sports drinks" research is conducted); in other words, under conditions that few kids of that age ever experience.

When I shared the results with Mansukhani, she was unconvinced: "This study doesn't prove that sports drinks are better at hydrating kids. The researcher's definition of superior 'hydration' seems to be mainly based on the fact that children drank more Capri-Sun. But we know the reason kids drank more is because they like the taste. To say a sports drink has a true hydration benefit, they would have to study a large number of kids, do a detailed evaluation to document dehydration, and show that the child's status improved with the sports drink." Mansukhani says that in the average child or adult's healthy diet, there is no role for sports drinks, and that water is best for hydration.[37]

The Processed-Food Conundrum: Nature Nourishes Best

Too often I hear nutrition advocates argue that when a company makes a change, even a less than perfect one, that's "a step in the right direction." As if food corporations have begun to "see the light" and, with a little coaxing, it's only a matter of time before they transform themselves into purveyors of truly healthy products. One colleague even admonished me for speaking out negatively about the PepsiCo Smart Spot, apparently worried that my public skepticism would discourage more "desirable" corporate behavior. But what my well-meaning colleagues fail to realize is that if companies can make money selling so-called healthier products, they will continue to do so, but once the nutriwashing marketing fails to generate sufficient revenue, it's game over. And truly healthy foods from nature do not generate sufficient profits for Big Food to continue making "steps in the right direction." Ultimately, any steps a food corporation takes will always be in the direction of more profit, an objective that has little to do with safeguarding public health.

Here's another line of reasoning I hear a lot: well, people are going to eat processed food anyway, so we should encourage companies to make those foods better. Such cynical reasoning doesn't cut it for me, either. As nutrition advocates, it's our job to be honest about what is optimally healthy, rather than meekly acquiesce to industry-supplied definitions. The argument that people aren't going to eat whole unprocessed foods becomes a self-fulfilling prophesy that is both condescending and immoral. Imagine if tobacco-control advocates argued that it's pointless to urge people to quit smoking because, well, they won't. Why is it any different when it comes to our expectations around getting people to change how they eat? Of course, ensuring that people have *access* to the right kinds of foods is an entirely different story. I am just saying that we shouldn't take it as a *given* that people are only going to eat processed foods. Also, accepting the status quo plays right into industry's rhetorical hands, allowing them to call the shots and control the debate.

In their wishful thinking, food companies would have us believe that doing away with obesity and other diet-related public health problems is simply a matter of encouraging people to exercise more and incorporate a few slightly less nutritionally odious products into their regular, "fun-for-you" dietary regimens. But in reality, solving the nation's health woes will take more much than magic-wand waving. Humans evolved on foods that came from nature, not a box or a can. Moreover, clean water supplies helped sustain human populations for eons prior to the industrial revolution. What comes out of most food factories today bears little resemblance to water or foods found in the natural world. Try as they might, the high-tech R&D laboratories of today's rich and powerful food corporations simply cannot improve on Mother Nature.

Indeed, whatever "health"-oriented innovations they dream up, the major packaged-food companies must continue—on pain of going out of business—to sell the American public a steady diet of highly processed products full of some combination of fat, sugar, and salt. Such concoctions of laboratory science will continue to be mechanically adulterated and infused with additives and chemicals that impart flavor, extend shelf life, or otherwise "enhance" them. Indeed, much of the corporate talk I hear related to obesity speaks glowingly of how food companies will invent techno-solutions by "creating" healthier food.

That nature has already taken care of this problem is of no interest to Big Food, since "value-added" processing allows manufacturers to charge inflated prices, generating revenue they can then reinvest to expand market share and accumulate more profit. In the end, these basic precepts of market economics are the piper that calls the tune. Because multinational food conglomerates must remain competitive on a global scale, they simply cannot market the truly healthful foods that nature has already provided for us.

What, then, are processed-food manufacturers supposed to do when public health experts and nutrition advocates concerned about Americans' dismal diet start pointing fingers in their direction? Obviously, closing up shop or directing people to their local farmers' markets are not appealing options. However, developing new industrial foods and spinning them as "healthful" is. Such "better-for-you" products are aimed at convincing both policy makers and "concerned moms" that industry is dutifully exercising its civic responsibility to provide "alternatives," so really, what is all the fuss about?

But in the long run, we cannot rely on the food industry to reformulate, repackage, or relabel its way out of the morass of public health problems that it has helped create. Regardless of how much "whole grain" they add to Chips Ahoy cookies, companies like Kraft cannot provide us with the kind of optimal nutrition found in fresh fruits and vegetables. No matter how hard they try to convince you otherwise, the food and beverage industries have only their own best interests at heart. The rest is just a bunch of nutriwash.

6

"Responsible Marketing" to Kids

The Lunchables Brigade is racing to the scene of a large party where routine lunch is on the menu.[1]

—"Advergame" for kids on Kraft Foods Web site

I must confess that I don't have children of my own. But I still care about what kids eat. And I especially care about how children are being exploited by major food companies. The eating habits that children form early in life predict how they will eat for the rest of their lives, which in turn has a lasting impact on their health.

Marketing to kids is big business. Kids are spending more of their own money at younger ages. They also influence a substantial proportion of the total sales of certain foods, including salty snacks, soft drinks, frozen pizza, and cold cereals.[2] The problem of excessive junk food marketing to kids is well documented by other authors and consumer groups.³ In recent years, the issue has taken center stage in the national debate surrounding the causes of the childhood obesity epidemic. Also, children are increasingly experiencing health problems previously seen only in adults, such as Type 2 diabetes and early signs of heart disease.

With children being bombarded with forty thousand commercials a year, combined with an ever-increasing onslaught of high-tech vehicles to reach kids anytime and anywhere, parents and professionals alike are saying enough is enough. (Schools are another area of great concern, which we will cover in Chapter 10.) Young children have not yet developed the cognitive ability to even realize they are being marketed to; they cannot understand what's called "persuasive intent." For all of these reasons and more, prominent professional organizations, including the American Academy of Pediatrics, the American Psychological Association, and the American Public Health Association are calling upon the federal government to intervene and protect children from predatory marketing by food corporations.

Feeling the heat, food companies that heavily market products to children have gone on the defensive. They insist that "self-regulation" rather than government oversight is sufficient, and have forged their own policies of "responsible" marketing to children. The goal is to contain the threat of government regulation and lawsuits, and especially to promote good public relations. But underneath the PR veneer lie little more than empty promises and a dizzying array of loopholes and corporate spin. The result is food marketing to kids that is more confusing than ever.

Confusing Kids with Advertising

If you're one of the many adults baffled by the endless hyped-up nutrition messages put out by the food industry, just imagine what that cacophony must sound like to a child. Kristen Harrison, a professor of speech communication at the University of Illinois at Urbana-Champaign, has researched how marketing contributes to children's confusion about nutrition: "Child television viewers are bombarded with health claims in television advertising. Given the plentitude of advertisements on television touting the health benefits of even the most nutritionally bankrupt of foods, child viewers are likely to become confused about which foods are in fact healthy."[4]

Harrison is especially concerned about the marketing of foods lacking in nutrients that children need to grow. Products with deceptively healthy-sounding labels such as "diet" and "fat-free," for example, make it hard for kids to understand the difference between nutritious, growth-promoting foods and those that may contribute to becoming overweight. Harrison's research also shows that whether kids are watching children's or adult programming, they are exposed to ads for unhealthy foods. She concludes that "television in general seems to be a source of nutritional misinformation, and children's exposure to television in general may increase their risk of becoming misinformed food consumers."[5]

Breakfast of Campaigners

A good example of the confusion so-called responsible marketing creates for kids occurred when the Children's Advertising Review Unit (CARU)—industry's own self-anointed "oversight" body—gave its blessing to an absurd ad campaign by General Mills, one of the top makers of children's cereals. In the wake of increasing criticism of sugary cereals, the company decided to portray itself as a champion of children's health with television ads dubbed "Choose Breakfast." Launched in June 2005, the campaign purports to "communicate the benefits of breakfast to children."[6] But can a company that boasts such candy-branded products as Reese's ' Puffs really get away with this?

While General Mills tried to lend an air of "public service" respectability by claming the campaign is "non-branded," the ten-second spots are suspiciously paired with twenty-second commercials for the company's kid-oriented cereals, including Lucky Charms, Cocoa Puffs, and Trix. Also, popular mascots such as the Trix rabbit and the Lucky Charms leprechaun appear in the ads to tout the benefits of physical activity—presumably to help kids work off all the sugar found in bowls of hearts, moons, stars, and clovers.

The company claims that it's not trying to promote its own cereals: the goal is simply to get kids to eat breakfast in the morning, Marybeth Thorsgaard, a General Mills spokeswoman, told the press. "We are advertising 'Choose Breakfast,'" she said. "We are not talking about cereal or a specific kind of breakfast."[7] In response, *Food Politics* author Marion Nestle was incredulous: "How can we possibly believe that? These companies don't do public service announcements. They have to be ads for their own cereals," she said.[8] Indeed, given the juxtaposition, how can children possibly be expected to distinguish between a Trix commercial and a supposed public service plug?

Moreover, the ads clearly violate CARU's own guidelines.

Ellen Fried, who teaches food law at New York University, says that CARU should have taken swift action to banish the ads, "but instead, they joined hands with General Mills by anointing their campaign. The company deftly sought preapproval and got even more."[9] Indeed, CARU director Elizabeth Lascoutx had nothing but praise for General Mills, quoted in the company's press release: "Ensuring that positive, nonbranded health messages like Choose Breakfast are being delivered to children is not only responsible, but commendable."[10] Fried was astonished by Lascoutx's pronouncement: "Either she didn't see the ads, didn't know they were being corrupted by General Mills' branded spots or isn't adequately applying the guidelines of the agency she directs, none of which is acceptable for an organization charged with protecting our children from unscrupulous advertisers."[11] The cozy relationship between CARU and General Mills is emblematic of the utter futility of self-regulation.

Coca-Cola: Marketing Myths and Loopholes

A major weakness of self-regulation is that it allows industry to limit the parameters of their responsibility. This puts them in a perfect position to overstate the benefits of their self-serving, loophole-ridden marketing policies. The Coca-Cola Company insists that it does not market its products to children under age twelve, which sounds great, but is it accurate? With public pressure over marketing to kids mounting, Coke announced in 2003: "In keeping with a policy that has been in place for more than half a century, the Coca-Cola Company and its local bottling partners do not aim or direct any marketing activity from any source to children under the age of twelve."[12]

American Coke Idol

While "no advertising to kids under twelve" may indeed mean that Coca-Cola doesn't advertise on cartoon shows aimed at young children, it also includes a huge exception for so-called mixed-audience television shows, which are viewed by both children and adults. Coke exploits this loophole through "product placement," where an item or corporate logo is embedded into programming for a more subliminal marketing effect than with commercials. The best example is *American Idol*—a top-rated show among children ages two to eleven—where Coca-Cola logos are emblazoned all over the set. According to Nielsen Media Research, during the 2004 season, Coca-Cola was the top overall sponsor of *American Idol*, with more than a staggering two thousand "branded occurrences."[13]

The company readily celebrates what it calls the show's "universal appeal," ranging from kids to older adults. David Raines, Coca-Cola's vice president of "integrated communications," told *USA Today* in 2002 when the show became an instant hit that "it's hard to find something that universal." Not to mention the value of scoring an end run around pesky federal rules that make product placement illegal on children's programming, but not on mixed shows. Further, Raines made the following eerie projection: "This is the future way we're going to have to communicate our brand."[14]

Coke-branded toys

Also, according to Coke: "Marketing or advertising for products bearing trademarks owned by the Coca-Cola Company, such as clothing, toys, novelties, and collectibles, are subject to these same guidelines."[15] And yet Coke-branded toys, including checker sets and cars, are aimed at children as young as age four. The company claims that as long as there are no commercials for these products, children are not being marketed to. So, because Coke gets to define the rules, they also get to decide when the rules are broken.

Coke's nonpolicy school policy

Coke also claims: "We will not promote our brands to children under twelve in schools and will respect their classroom as a commercial-free zone."[16] This statement is misleading at best.

Coca-Cola aggressively markets its products in schools to children of all ages, through exclusive "pouring rights" contracts. While the company points to its model guidelines that recommend soda not be sold in elementary school (the rules do permit sales in middle and high schools), the policy is voluntary and not enforced.[17] The Coke guidelines amount to little more than words on paper, because they don't bind the local bottlers who operate independently and actually contract with schools. That explains why a 2002 survey of Kentucky schools found 44 percent of elementary schools had vending machines.[18] Not coincidentally, as we will see, Coca-Cola has lobbied hard for four years running against state legislation designed to fix Kentucky's school vending problem.

Kraft Foods' Advertising Policy

When it comes to spinning itself as a responsible corporate

citizen where kids are concerned, Kraft Foods wins the prize hands down. It's no accident that Kraft is owned by Altria, which is also the parent company of tobacco giant Philip Morris. Kraft executives explain that they don't want to repeat the same "mistakes" of the tobacco wars. In other words, the company wants to avoid negative PR and protracted legal battles by being "part of the solution." That's why in January 2005, Kraft adopted a well-coordinated strategy for marketing to children. So what's wrong with that? Don't we want companies to curb their marketing practices toward children? Of course, but only if that's the actual result, rather than just corporate spin.

Timing is everything

Kraft's promise to scale back ads to children came on the very same day that the federal government released its updated 2005 Dietary Guidelines for Americans. The timing of Kraft's move was no coincidence. It was likely an attempt to (1) counteract the media's increasingly critical scrutiny of its nutritionally dubious products, and (2) piggyback on the government's announcement in hopes of aligning itself with the concept of healthy eating.

The announcement also came two weeks prior to the company's presentation for the Institute of Medicine (IOM) committee on food marketing to children. Kraft's timing was critical to being able to demonstrate to a prestigious government advisory body that self-regulation was working just fine, just in case any committee members might consider recommending congressional action.

Timing came in handy once again when Kraft's modified

marketing to kids policy (expanded to include Web sites) was announced in September 2005. Kraft's CEO himself, Roger Deromedi, made the big presentation, which was accompanied by the launch of several new, allegedly healthier products, including Whole Grain Chips Ahoy cookies, at California governor Arnold Schwarzenegger's invitation-only Summit on Health, Nutrition and Obesity.

Doing so earned Kraft a spot on the governor's "honor roll" of companies making significant "commitments" to solving the obesity problem—and a generous dose of free government PR to boot. Kraft's Deromedi also had a coveted seat on a panel of "leaders of change" at the event, which was heavily covered by both local and national media, including the *New York Times*.

ON TIMING OF KRAFT'S ANNOUNCEMENTS:

Government releases updated Dietary Guidelines	January 12, 2005
Kraft announces new advertising to kids' policy and Sensible Solutions Program	January 12, 2005
Industry forms Alliance for American Advertising (Kraft, General Mills, and Kellogg)	January 26, 2005
IOM Committee meeting on marketing to kids	January 27, 2005
Kraft announces expansion of policy to Web sites, introduces new "whole-grain" cookies, crackers	September 15, 2005
California Summit on Obesity (Kraft CEO recognized by governor on "honor roll")	September 15, 2005

Nutrition for kids, brought to you by Kraft

Kraft's marketing policy amounts to this: certain products, including original Kool-Aid, Oreo cookies, several Post children's cereals, and some varieties of Lunchables, will no longer be advertised to children ages six to eleven in TV, print, radio, and other media. However, other products aimed specifically at the six to eleven age group (Kraft says it already doesn't market its products to children under age six) will continue to be advertised, such as sugar-free Kool-Aid, ½ the Sugar Fruity Pebbles cereal (yes, that's really the name), and Chicken Dunks Lunchables Fun Pack. Kraft claims that these products offer "beneficial nutrients or a functional benefit" and are thus part of its new Sensible Solutions labeling program (discussed in Chapter 5).[19]

Why does Kraft get to define what is and isn't healthy? Has Kool-Aid suddenly become healthier for kids now that it comes in a sugar-free version that uses the artificial sweetener aspartame—which has been linked to numerous health problems, including seizures, migraines, and brain tumors,[20] versus the tooth-rotting sugar found in the original formula?

Also, Kraft's criteria for their frozen meals, which includes Lunchables, allows up to 600 calories, which for a kid, health policy consultant and endocrinologist Dr. Renu Mansukhani says, is likely to be far too high. "Only kids who do more than an hour of vigorous activity daily should be eating 600 calories at one sitting." Also, Kraft's allowable range for salt is 480–960 milligrams of sodium. Mansukhani says that 960 milligrams "seems like an awfully high upper limit for a 'healthy' line of products."[21]

The Sensible Solutions line of Lunchables includes "Pepperoni Flavored Sausage Pizza," a bad sign already. (I have no idea what "pepperoni flavored sausage" means; such factory concoctions were never available at my neighborhood Italian pizzeria growing up in New York; we had either sausage or pepperoni, why would you flavor one with the other?) This product contains 450 calories (a large amount for a child) and 34 grams of sugar along with 600 milligrams of sodium (both high levels for a child). Mansukhani says she is not a big fan of any Lunchables. "I am a parent and I know parents need quick solutions for packing lunch, but there are lots of other non-processed and healthy items, such as yogurt and fruit. Sure, kids like pizza, but pizza can be made in a healthier way than in Lunchables without a lot of effort," she said.[22]

Such do-it-yourself ideas won't help Kraft, which has a major financial stake in Lunchables, especially the pizza varieties, which have traditionally been best sellers, accounting for 30 percent of Lunchables' sales. Moreover, the Lunchables line has an 85 percent share of the $750 million market for prepackaged kids' lunches. But increasing competition and a declining reputation among parents meant that sales increased by just 1.5 percent in 2004–2005.[23] That explains in part why Kraft is so eager to reformulate to win back parents.

The ad dollars shell game

Besides the nutritional dubiousness, what gets lost in most press accounts is that Kraft doesn't plan to reduce overall advertising expenditures for marketing aimed at kids; rather, it will simply change the way these funds are allocated. This crucial detail is not hidden; it's right there in the company press release, which clearly states that the firm "will continue to advertise its full portfolio of products in television, radio, and print media seen principally by parents and all-family audiences" and "market its products through means such as packaging, Web sites, and in-store promotions."[24] In other words, Kraft will simply shift some of its budget for advertising unhealthy, "general-audience" products (e.g., Oreos) over to marketing slightly less unhealthy products (e.g., "½ the Sugar" Fruity Pebbles) directly to kids, in certain media. (Are you with me?)

Even some commentators in the business community recognize the Kraft move as relatively insignificant. For example, David Kiley of *BusinessWeek* notes that the Kraft "move seems, at best, to be on the margins of the debate. The food items that won't be pushed on TV programs will still be on the Internet, in magazines, and outdoor media aimed at the same under-twelve audience. And the cartoon characters will still be all over the packaging when children go shopping with Mom and Dad. Furthermore, media experts say those kids are increasingly logging on to the Net and watching recorded TV via DVDs and TiVo, anyway."[25]

Tricia Wilber, senior vice president of ad sales and promotion for ABC Cable Networks Group, told *MediaWeek* that she doesn't anticipate Kraft getting out of the kid marketing business anytime soon: "It isn't that Kraft is pulling out of kids, it is what they are advertising that will be different. From our perspective, we are still trying to figure out what dollars are working, but we feel it will be pretty healthy" (as in, "healthy" profits). Jim Perry, Nickelodeon's senior vice president of ad sales, agrees that advertisers like Kraft are just coming up with new ways to market new products to children.[26]

We didn't mean all Web sites: the advergaming loophole

"Advergaming," another important form of marketing to children, involves the incorporation of ad messages into free video games on children's Web sites. While Kraft's January 2005 policy announcement avoided any mention of Web sites, the company later (probably under pressure) decided to include them under its marketing to kids policy. So in September 2005, it declared: "By the end of 2006, only products that meet Kraft's Sensible Solution nutrition standards will appear on Kraft Web sites that primarily reach children ages six–eleven."[27]

But the impact is less than it might seem. First, note the convenient and potentially gaping loophole that Kraft grants itself with the qualifier "primarily." Obviously kid-friendly Web sites target a range of ages. This could mean that if a Kraft Web site is visited by children 51 percent of whom are over age eleven, no changes are made; and of course, children of any age can access such sites.

But why make the announcement more than a year before the policy's implementation? When I asked Mark Berlind, then Kraft's executive vice president for global corporate affairs, to explain the delay, he told me the company needed the time to make the Web changes and develop more Sensible Solutions products aimed at kids.[28] Why not wait until the policy is in place to go public? Or if Kraft was really concerned for kids' welfare and couldn't wait to share its epiphany, why not shut down the sites altogether until the company is ready with the new and allegedly improved products?

In the meantime, Kraft Web sites such as "NabiscoWorld" and "Postopia" are chock-full of games and promotions that young kids are sure to love, promoting Oreos, Chips Ahoy, and the rest of Kraft's non–Sensible Solution products. Here is how the company itself describes these sites: "Kraft also offers information, games, snack ideas, and more to children of all ages through Nabiscoworld.com and Postopia.com."[29] Just what kids need: "snack ideas" from the creators of Cheez Whiz, Mallomars, and Cool Whip.

A particularly sinister example of advergaming is the "Pizza and Treatza" game featured on Kraft's Lunchables Web site. "The Lunchables Brigade's mission," kids are told, is to "fight routine lunch."[30] Even the industry-friendly Children's Advertising Review Unit (CARU) said the Lunchables Brigade ad campaign was out of bounds. In a report issued in November 2005, CARU "discussed concerns regarding the depiction of Lunchables in the context of a balanced meal as well as potential issues of product denigration." Specifically, CARU admonished Kraft for depicting the Lunchables Brigade as "coming to the rescue of children who have been provided with a homemade lunch of what the Brigade describes as "leftover chicken legs—ouch."[31] In response, Kraft "agreed to keep in mind CARU's concerns regarding product denigration as it develops future advertising."[32] (Last I checked, the Web site remains unchanged.)

We didn't mean cartoons: the character loophole

Kraft's marketing to children is also noteworthy for its liberal deployment of kid-friendly characters such as Batman, the Flintstones (which boasts its own cereal line), the Hulk, and many Disney favorites. Nothing in Kraft's children's advertising policy suggests any intention to abandon this tactic, meaning that parents are still subject to nagging when kids see their favorite characters adorning Kraft products on supermarket shelves. I picked up a bag of Cheese Nips endorsed by characters from Nickelodeon's hit show *Fairly OddParents*. The package looks more like an ad for the TV program than a container of food. The show is second in popularity only to *SpongeBob SquarePants* (which endorses other Kraft products) with kids aged two to eleven; so much for not marketing to kids under age six. Also, Kraft hawks five star-studded varieties of its infamous macaroni and cheese, all of which conveniently qualify for the company's Sensible Solutions flag ensuring continued marketing to kids:[33]

- Kraft Macaroni & Cheese *The Fairly OddParents*
- Kraft Macaroni & Cheese *SpongeBob SquarePants*
- Kraft Macaroni & Cheese *Rugrats*
- Kraft Macaroni & Cheese *Scooby Doo*
- Supermac & Cheese *Spiderman*

We didn't mean sales: the school loophole

In view of the recent clamor to get junk food out of schools, Kraft has taken great pains to demonstrate what a great a corporate citizen it is here as well. While Kraft claims it "has eliminated advertising and promotion in schools," there's just one little catch: its products are still *sold* in schools. Remarkably, the company readily acknowledges this contradiction, explaining that it will only sell products that meet the Sensible Solutions criteria.[34] It is utterly disingenuous to promise to stop in-school promotion but still *sell* products in school. How can the sale of food not count as promotion? What if you walked into a school store and measured the amount of square footage taken up by packaged foods such as Kraft's ubiquitous cookie brands? Food packaging is designed by highly skilled marketing experts, and kids' products are especially eye-catching.

Kraft's Loophole of Confusion: The Branding Problem

A major problem with Kraft's policy of "shifting the mix" of products over to its self-defined Sensible Solutions product line is that in every case, the product packaging for the "non-advertised" products looks virtually identical to the new Sensible Solutions products. Of course, this problem is magnified when you look at the world through the eyes of a young child: in colors and shapes.

For example, what child do you know who is going to ask for "sugar-free Kool-Aid," as opposed to just "Kool-Aid"? Kraft is fully aware of this problem, and yet at the time of this writing—well over a year after the January 2005 press release—it has done nothing about it. When the company made the announcement, Kraft's vice president, Mark Berlind, said that Kraft intended to make sure any ads directed at young children would "look and feel different" from those created for their less healthful counterparts.[35] I heard him repeat this concern in September 2005 at a media event on obesity, but I still heard no plan of action. While it's nice that the company acknowledges the problem, I am having a hard time imagining exactly what sort of fix Kraft has in mind, given the high-stakes competition of the lucrative children's market: plain black text on white packaging?

The reason this is important is that Kraft isn't going to stop *making* the non–Sensible Solutions products that are aimed at kids; it just isn't going to market them in certain ways anymore. The unhealthy products remain on store shelves. So when a child walks down the cereal aisle and sees two boxes that look virtually identical but one says "½ the Sugar Fruity Pebbles" and the other says simply "Fruity Pebbles," she is likely to nag her parent for the full-sugar version, despite having seen ads for its less sugary counterpart. The question then becomes: what is the actual impact of Kraft's marketing policy on children?

Sensible Lunchables

One of the more fun parts of my job is constantly learning about and being amazed by food-industry creativity. Do you have any idea how many Lunchables varieties Kraft manufactures? Would you believe fifty-six? Now, guess how many qualify for the corporate Sensible Solutions seal. While the company's R&D department is probably scrambling to come up with more, as of March 2006, only six varieties of Sensible Solutions Lunchables existed, or roughly 11 percent of the entire product line. Those six "nutritious" varieties are:

- Lunchables Chicken Dunks
- Lunchables BBQ Chicken Shake-Ups
- Lunchables Nacho Cheese Chicken Shake-Ups
- Lunchables Extra Cheesy Pizza
- Lunchables Pepperoni Flavored Sausage Pizza
- Lunchables Pizza & Treatza

I visited my neighborhood Safeway grocery store to get some idea of the scope of the problem in a real-life setting. Sure enough, in the refrigerated section I counted eighteen distinct varieties of Lunchables. Of those, four contained the Sensible Solution flag.

Anyway, why not just market these products to parents? Dr. Mansukhani says that if Kraft's Sensible Solutions products are truly healthier, then they should be marketed to parents and not to kids, especially since companies are saying that what children eat is the parents' responsibility. "The kids they are marketing these products to are not old enough to make these decisions. The kid sees big Kool-Aid guy and that's all they will see."[36]

One Krafty PR Machine

One of the most irritating aspects of Kraft's marketing to kids policy is how favorably their corporate fanfare was received by the mainstream media, which dutifully furthered the company's PR efforts. An exaggerated headline in the *Chicago Tribune*, for example, read: "Kraft Will No Longer Aim Ads for Unhealthy Snacks at Youngsters."[37] Others were similarly effusive: "Kraft Takes Lead in Responsibility"[38] (*Advertising Age* editorial) and "Obesity Fears Prompt Kraft to Stop Targeting Children with Junk Food Ads"[39] (*Financial Times of London*). (In contrast, the *New York Times*, *Washington Post*, and *Wall Street Journal* ran more measured headlines.)

To this day, countless newspaper stories continue to erroneously report that Kraft has "stopped marketing unhealthy food to kids"—or words to that effect—even when, as we have seen, its policy hardly rises to the level of a sweeping ban on children's marketing. Of course, this is exactly what Kraft was counting on: lazy reporters who reinforce the company's own sound bite framing, which is designed to make the move sound much better than it is.

You Gotta Fight for Your Right to Advertise

Major food corporations like to have it both ways. On the one hand, they want to claim an inviolable right to market their products any way they please. On the other hand, they urgently want to position themselves as "part of the solution."

An excellent example of this came less than two weeks after Kraft's January 2005 announcement of its new children's ad policy when the food giant paid $25,000 to join other major food companies and ad agencies to create a new lobbying group called the Alliance for American Advertising.[40] Kraft and fellow members General Mills and Kellogg are the top three advertisers of packaged food to kids, with combined annual spending on children's ads approaching $380 million in the United States alone.

Other alliance founders include the American Association of Advertising Agencies and the Grocery Manufacturers Association, two powerful trade associations in their own right. The alliance's stated purpose is to defend the industry's First Amendment right to advertise to children and to promote self-regulation as an alternative to government restrictions.[41]

Consuming Kids author Susan Linn is appalled at this industry power grab: "Marketing to children is not an absolute right. Food companies and the advertising industry should be thinking about their responsibilities to children, not about their 'right' to exploit them."[42] What better evidence do we need that "industry leaders" such as Kraft cannot be trusted to self regulate than their forming such a lobbying coalition?

Since its announcement, the Kraft ad policy toward kids has been a persistent thorn in my side. I often find myself trying to undo the exaggerated positive PR spin that too many others have bestowed on Kraft. Especially troubling has been the upbeat reaction that Kraft's advertising policy has enjoyed among some public health advocates who should know better. It just takes digging a little deeper to reveal that Kraft's campaign is rife with loopholes that promise to create more, not less, confusion for the "little consumers" it targets.

Playing Tricks with a Powerful Sponge

Few children's cartoon characters ever reach the level of celebrity stardom and marketing domination as Nickelodeon's SpongeBob SquarePants. Estimates are that seventy-five marketers manufacture a whopping ten thousand SpongeBob-themed products, generating $25 million in licensing fees for corporate parent Viacom in 2002 alone.[43] But with nutrition and children's advocates voicing louder concerns over tie-ins with such nutrient-deficient foods as Kellogg's Pop-Tarts, Nabisco (Kraft) CheeseNips, and Burger King kids' meals, the children's cable network decided it is was time to salvage SpongeBob's

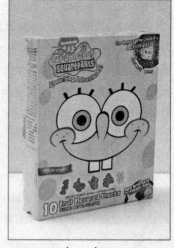

Luring Kids with Cartoons

reputation. In classic two-faced corporate style, however, Nick-elodeon didn't actually stop any of the junk food tie-ins with the happy sponge, but rather the company just added some window dressing in hopes of silencing its critics. While Nick might now appear to be only looking out for your child's best interests, the company is not fooling everyone.

As *BusinessWeek* commentator David Kiley explains, "SpongeBob and his fellow cartoon stars are being used to pro-mote better eating habits and exercise by way of programming, public-service style ads, and Web site content," but Nick-elodeon is simultaneously benefiting from the royalties derived from SpongeBob and Dora the Explorer touting junk food:

> To make the scene more confusing for kids and par-ents, SpongeBob, which drives about $1 billion a year in licensed goods, is now featured on Kraft Macaroni & Cheese and Nabisco Fruit Snacks in new "Nicktri-tional" labels, doling out advice such as drinking lots of water and playing games like soccer for exercise. Nick-tritional labeling is an idea driven by Nickelodeon, anx-ious to avoid becoming a lightning rod for childhood obesity. Nick spokesman David Bittler admits that its efforts, like SpongeBob touting healthy living habits, are sending mixed signals.[44]

Bittler says that Nick has been trying to get advertisers to use its cartoon characters on healthier offerings, but it's been a tough sell. Apparently, it doesn't pay to license expensive cartoon char-acters to advertise healthful stuff on kids' programming because the audience doesn't respond. Kiley quotes one food company executive, who asked not to be identified: "I can't write a return-on-investment business case—unless it's purely for public relations—for advertising fruit or whole-grain crackers on Nick or any other kids' program."[45] This, in a nutshell, is precisely why we cannot expect corporate kid-friendly marketing to truly promote healthy eating; it just doesn't pay.

Moreover, Susan Linn says that using cartoon characters to sell any food to children is harmful because it teaches them to choose food based on packaging, as opposed to nutritional value or taste. She's also concerned about mixed messages: "Branded broccoli and star-studded spinach aren't going to make a dent in the problem of childhood obesity if children continue to be bombarded with media icons selling all kinds of junk food as well. I don't hear Nickelodeon saying they are going to remove SpongeBob SquarePants from packages of ice cream, cookies, and candy."[46]

It's a SpongeBob life

Now, it may appear that SpongeBob is just an innocent cartoon; what harm can he possibly do? But consider what turning the cute marine creature into a major marketing vehicle has meant for many children, who now exist in a world of twenty-four-hour SpongeBob reality. Life in such a universe means waking up in SpongeBob bedding in a room with SpongeBob wallpaper and SpongeBob furniture; eating SpongeBob Pop-Tarts for breakfast; going to school with a SpongeBob lunchbox and SpongeBob backpack; wearing a SpongeBob T-shirt; playing a SpongeBob video game after school; covering up a scrape with a SpongeBob Band-Aid; bathing with a SpongeBob towel and SpongeBob shower curtain; eating

SpongeBob macaroni and cheese for dinner; brushing your teeth with a SpongeBob toothbrush and SpongeBob toothpaste; and climbing back into your SpongeBob bed and SpongeBob pajamas. Where does it all end?

Stop the Insanity

If we care about children's overall well-being, do we really want to perpetuate rampant commercialism aimed at kids by calling for *more* characters to promote eating the right kinds of foods, when natural hunger signals, the pleasure of eating, and role modeling should suffice? In other words, the same motivations that drive (or should) adult healthy eating behavior.

It may sound petty to argue that the solution does not lie in using cartoon characters on healthy foods. Indeed, there is a split among advocates on this issue. Some believe that it's perfectly fine to use cartoons to market healthy products such as spinach and carrots to children under the theory of whatever works. Others argue that it's still harmful and confusing. Why should we worry about this? If we only narrowly confine the issue to the use of cartoon characters (and other child-friendly practices) to market junk food, we miss the potential harm caused by commercialism more generally.[47]

Another reason it's important to avoid speaking about "marketing healthy foods to kids" is that it plays right into the hands of industry. At every government meeting on the subject, the leading food corporations have gone to great lengths to extol the virtues of their current and future plans to market so-called healthier products to children, with nary a word spoken about how they are curbing the marketing of junk food products. This frame helps industry by keeping corporations in the driver's seat: if we are asking for companies to market healthier foods to children (and to use cartoon characters and other child-friendly promotions), in the current self-regulatory environment, this means that the companies themselves get to define what constitutes "healthier products" and how those allegedly healthier products get marketed—which is exactly what is happening.

It is critical that advocates, policy makers, and the public not be fooled by industry pronouncements of responsible marketing. The devil is truly in the details. We should not rely on the food industry to set public health policy, and especially not when it comes to marketing to children. The corporate imperative to maximize profits will always ultimately run roughshod over the ethical obligation to safeguard children's health and well-being.

Ten Tips for Critically Evaluating Corporate Self-regulatory Ad Policies:

1. Always read the original corporate press release and don't rely on media or other secondhand accounts of what the policy says. Also, be sure to read the release to the end, where the devilish details can be buried.

2. Ask: what's the timing of the announcement? Is the company trying to take advantage of some other major public relations opportunity?

3. Look for dates: when is the policy supposed to go into effect? Sometimes the policy is announced long before actual implementation. Be wary of phrases like "as current commitments expire" or "phase out," which

could mean the company has bought advertising for months into the future.

4. Spot the loopholes: what exactly does the policy accomplish? What are the specific advertising media and age ranges the policy covers? What's left out of the policy and why? Consider the *numerous* forms of marketing and not just TV commercials. Other methods include product placement, cross promotions, movie tie-ins, advergaming, and package displays.

5. Look for sneaky qualifiers that might water down the impact. For example, Kraft's policy says it applies to media "primarily viewed" by children ages six to eleven, which is another way of saying that mixed media are still fair game.

6. Don't be fooled by self-aggrandizing words like *initiative* or *commitment* or even *policy*. Companies like to make their press releases sound much more important than they really are.

7. What's the oversight mechanism? Who's making sure the company follows through with its promises? Where is the accountability?

8. Look for any self-defined and dubious nutrition criteria, such as products that make up for less sugar with artificial sweeteners.

9. Look for the policy's impact, if any, in other countries. If it's only effective in the United States, this could either mean the company doesn't market as much abroad, or, more likely, that the U.S. climate currently poses more of a public relations threat. In other words, the company is just putting out fires.

10. Don't believe anybody else's interpretation of a corporate ad policy, even among public health advocates and especially not most media. Always do your own critical analysis and come to your own conclusions.

Exposing
Government Complicity

First, we have to continue to work hard to spread the gospel of personal responsibility.[1]
—Tommy Thompson, (former) Secretary of Health and Human Services

While it makes sense that the food industry's profit motive to sell more food would bring it into direct conflict with public health, it's less intuitive that the federal government would also fail to act in the public's best interests. And yet, when it comes to solving the nation's epidemic of diet-related diseases, Uncle Sam is more aligned with Big Food than with the citizens it's supposed to represent. Understanding the links between industry and government rhetoric is critical to being able to spot it when it happens and not be fooled.[2]

Hiding the Truth about Nutrition

Every five years, the U.S. Department of Agriculture (USDA) releases its Dietary Guidelines for Americans. Based on the latest nutrition science, each new edition is eagerly anticipated by a media that treats its findings as the gold standard on which foods are best to eat to stay healthy. But while the dietary guidelines purport to be a "primary source of dietary health information for policy makers, nutrition educators, and health providers," they really reflect how much more closely aligned the federal government is with industry than with the general public.

The 2005 Dietary Guidelines were touted as having the strongest recommendations yet, but what went unsaid explains why Americans continue to be left in the dark when it comes to healthy eating. The new guidelines focus heavily on weight loss and getting regular exercise. (Remember, these are supposed to be *dietary* rules, not overall healthful-living tips.) The problem with the weight and exercise slant is that it emphasizes individual behavior while skirting the crucial public-policy questions related to which foods to eat and which ones to avoid.

In fact, when it comes to food, the dietary guidelines tell only part of the story—the politically expedient part. Under the heading "Food Groups to Encourage" are fruits, vegetables, and whole grains. These foods are glaringly deficient in the diets of most Americans, many of whom don't even know what a whole grain is or where to find one. You can't go to the supermarket and ask the shop clerk for the whole-grain aisle, but you can easily find the potato-chip aisle or the cookie aisle or the soda aisle.

Americans have become accustomed to eating highly processed foods that come in a package—the antithesis of whole foods that come from nature. The very definition of food has been transformed by industry, yet the dietary guidelines don't reflect that. If they did, it would be a major threat to a $500-billion-a-year processed-foods industry, whose voice is heard loud and clear in Washington, especially when it comes to what is said in the dietary guidelines. Something else the federal government isn't telling us is how to avoid harmful trans fats. Dr. Carlos Camargo of the Harvard Medical School and a member of the dietary guidelines committee said he was "disappointed" that the experts' unanimous recommendation to limit trans fats to 1 percent of calories was completely omitted from the final document.[3] Instead, we are told to simply "limit intake" of trans fat.

Why the change? *Food Politics* author Marion Nestle explains: "Trans fat was left vague because otherwise they would have to say where trans fats *are*—in processed foods."[4] In wording that Nestle calls "incomprehensible," the consumer-friendly guidelines brochure recommends that you "look for foods low in saturated fats and trans fats"—the two most common artery-clogging fats in the supermarket. Why would the government tell you to "look for" foods that you really should avoid altogether? Because it cannot say: don't eat too many of the major sources of saturated fats: meat, cheese, milk, and eggs. Nor could Uncle Sam tell us to avoid the main sources of trans fats: fried and baked goods such as chips, cakes, and cookies. That would ruffle too many industry feathers.

Some nutritionists were understandably pleased with the

government's sugar recommendation. That the sugar industry complained so loudly was certainly a good sign. Yet, part of the advice is simply to choose beverages with "little added sugars"—still pretty fuzzy language. Keeping the wording as vague as possible is good for big business. Is it any wonder that so many people are still confused about how to eat?

MyPyramid, Our Problem

Four months later, in April 2005, the federal government revealed its much-anticipated revision of the "Food Guide Pyramid"—that peculiar icon of nutrition advice that adorns cereal boxes and not much else. While the dietary guidelines are the written recommendations for how we should eat, the pyramid is a pictorial representation of the nutrition rules. According to the USDA's own surveys, most people (80 percent) recognize the triangular graphic, but only a sobering 2 to 4 percent actually follow its principles.[5]

To try to fix this problem, the agriculture department set out to create a new and improved version. In typical Washington style, the job was outsourced to the mega-PR firm Porter Novelli International. While past clients have included the likes of McDonald's and the Snack Food Association, the company promised there would be no conflict of interest.

So what did U.S. taxpayers get for their $2.5 million? Reactions from nutrition experts to the curious graphic—featuring little more than a few variously colored triangular segments alongside a stick figure climbing stairs—have been swift and unequivocal: the new "MyPyramid" is certainly no better and may even be worse than the old version. With all of the dietary details now available only via the Web site, buried deep among countless pages to click through, who on earth is going to bother to take the time?

The very name MyPyramid tells us the government is placing all responsibility for good nutrition squarely with you and me. Never mind those pesky government subsidies and tax breaks to big agribusiness and food manufacturers that make unhealthy food so cheap and ubiquitous. Thank goodness Uncle Sam has created a Web site to counter all that.

At a press conference unveiling the new pyramid, USDA Secretary Mike Johanns shared the stage with fitness guru Denise Austin. Introduced by Johanns as a "wife and mother," Austin, overflowing with energy, implored reporters to join her in a stretching routine. That the federal government's unveiling of a $2.5 million dietary educational tool was reduced to a Jane Fonda video was embarrassing to say the least.

But more insidiously, MyPyramid's emphasis on activity plays right into the food industry's hands. As we have seen, an important way that industry deflects blame for incessantly promoting unhealthy products is to point to the nation's couch potato tendencies. With MyPyramid, government officially adopted the food industry's argument that exercise is the real answer to the nation's health woes.

Of course exercise is important, but so are other healthy behaviors, such as getting enough sleep. If one side of the pyramid shows someone walking up stairs to emphasize the importance of exercise, why doesn't the other side show someone lying down to illustrate the importance of rest? Simply because poor sleep habits, unlike poor exercise habits, are unlikely targets for the food industry's blame game.

Let the Co-optation Begin

Because government announcements and policy statements garner a tremendous amount of press coverage, they serve as an important way for industry to help direct the nation's nutrition dialogue.

The major food companies' rush to embrace the new pyramid was a clear indication of just how friendly the scheme is to their interests. For example, on the same day as the government press conference, cereal boxes depicted on General Mills' Web site already contained the new image. "We want to help communicate these important messages by using some of the best real estate there is," boasted John Haugen of General Mills. "The cereal box is one of the most-read items in the home. With cereal consumed in 93 percent of American households, this is a powerful step forward in nutrition education," he said.[6] But the new graphic doesn't contain any actual information. And "reading" the food pyramid while downing a bowl of Lucky Charms isn't exactly what most nutritionists would call either sound education or a recommended dietary practice.

Just two days after MyPyramid's release, snack food and beverage giant PepsiCo jumped in to offer its own congratulations to Uncle Sam. In an ad in *USA Today*, the company declared itself in profound agreement with MyPyramid's emphasis on energy balance as a key concept in maintaining health. As mentioned earlier, "energy balance" is industry's subtle way of promoting its oversimplified calories-in/calories-out message. Conveniently, this formula says nothing about the vacant nutritional content of the calories. And if you're an image-conscious food maker, keeping the damning facts about your products hush-hush is a high priority.

On the same day, a press release from the Grocery Manufacturers Assocation (GMA) proudly announced plans to promote the new pyramid to students, teachers, and families. The trade group also took credit for the old icon's 80 percent recognition rate, saying it is "due, in part, to the efforts of the food and beverage industry,"[7] even though it wasn't so interested in taking credit for the fact that 96 to 98 percent of people don't follow it.[8]

In September 2005, the USDA (apparently needing a few more months to work out the kinks) unveiled "MyPyramid for Kids," chock-full of games and other entertainment of dubious educational value. Not missing a beat, the GMA introduced, on the very same day, a new curriculum designed to teach children about the special version of MyPyramid designed just for them. According to the GMA, "The new educational materials will be used by approximately 58,000 educators who reach more than four million students in grades 4–6."[9] But here's the kicker: "Recognizing that USDA has limited resources to promote MyPyramid, GMA identified grade schools as an area in which the private sector could help extend the government's nutrition message." GMA also pledged to translate its materials into Spanish and to distribute materials for free in "high-Hispanic populations." How ironic. The lobbying group that has fought against improving school nutrition policy in every state in the nation is going to distribute watered-down educational materials to bilingual kids in poor neighborhoods. Maybe if GMA and its members would stop marketing its diabetes-causing foods to "high-Hispanic populations," the kids wouldn't need any pamphlets.

Small Thinking, Small Steps

When it comes to poorly conceived nutrition-education campaigns emanating from Washington, the food pyramid has plenty of company. In March 2004, the Department of Health and Human Services (HHS) launched the Healthy Lifestyles and Disease Prevention Initiative. The campaign "encourages American families to take small, manageable steps within their current lifestyle—versus drastic changes—to ensure effective, long-term weight control."[10] It features (what else?) a Web site (www.smallstep.gov), where HHS Secretary Tommy Thompson explains that people don't need to resort to "extreme measures"—such as following a diet fad or joining a gym—to lose weight. Tips include such bold and original ideas as taking the stairs instead of an escalator.

Public health experts immediately questioned the campaign's effectiveness. For example, the Center for Science in the Public Interest called it "more talk and no real help" for millions of Americans.[11] Former U.S. surgeon general David Satcher said that he had "no objection to small steps," but insisted that "there also need to be big steps."[12]

The campaign also includes bizarre public service ads. One shows boys playing on a beach discovering a human belly and another features shoppers finding a double chin in a grocery store. Several surreal print ads focus on close-up shots of heavy stomachs, thighs, and buttocks and show how they might slim down as their owners get more active. There's a bus ad in my neighborhood that features a close-up picture of a largish woman's hip and thigh. (She's wearing a bathing suit.) I had to look closely to see what it was about. Is this image supposed to be my incentive to eat right and exercise? The message is elusive and offensive, not to mention a waste of taxpayer money.

March 2004 was a busy time for Uncle Sam in "tackling" the obesity problem. That month the Food and Drug Administration (FDA) also released its own "innovative" strategy, aimed at driving home the groundbreaking scientific discovery that "calories count." The report by the FDA's Obesity Working Group recommended that food makers place dietary advice on packages, such as, "To manage your weight, balance the calories you eat with your physical activity; have a carrot, not the carrot cake; or have cherry yogurt, not cherry pie."[13] So, in its wisdom, the FDA has told manufacturers to label its products to tell people to eat healthy, nonmanufactured foods like carrots—which normally come from the earth without labels or packaging. Does anyone review this stuff?

The FDA's "calories count" report is yet another example of tax dollars being squandered on toothless recommendations, with a focus on education and personal responsibility that suits industry just fine. But that was nothing compared to what I witnessed at a high-profile conference just two months later.

Tommy Thompson's Personal Responsibility Solution

In June 2004, *Time* magazine and ABC News cohosted a "summit on obesity" in historic Williamsburg, Virginia. The event was touted as "drawing together leaders across sectors and disciplines . . . to advance knowledge and focus attention on what can be done to turn this epidemic around."[14] The two-day conference featured a stellar lineup of expert speakers, more than 600 attendees, and, of course, lots of media opportunities. Among the high-profile presenters was Tommy Thompson, then U.S. secretary of health and human services and, not coincidentally, a man with zero background in public health.

In his keynote address, Thompson emphasized the seriousness of the obesity problem, noting that "America's eating habits and lack of physical activity are literally killing us, and they're killing us at records levels." Outlining his vision for solutions, Thompson wasted no time placing individual accountability front and center: "We have to do it ourselves," he said jovially, calling upon conference participants to "go out and spread the gospel of personal responsibility."

Thompson went on to explain how he had been meeting with food-industry leaders, urging them to make changes. Despite some initial resistance, Thompson claimed, food companies were becoming increasingly responsive, and he heaped glowing praise upon them for their alleged newfound altruism.

Thompson included Kraft, Coca-Cola, PepsiCo, and McDonald's on his list of companies committed to taking positive steps. He lauded Coca-Cola for "promising to end exclusive contracting in schools."[15] One problem: Coca-Cola never said that and never ended this practice. Instead, in 2001, the company released a voluntary policy that doesn't cover the local bottlers that contract with schools.[16] In other words, it was just a PR move, and Thompson fell for it.

Thompson also singled out McDonald's for its "conscientious" initiatives, including its new "Balanced Lifestyles Platform," as well as its decision to serve more "low-carb" options. (The secretary's glee over the growing prevalence of nutritionally dubious "low-carb" menu options was especially troubling—he referenced this "good news" more than once.) Then, just when I thought things couldn't get much worse, for some inexplicable reason, he took questions from the audience. Most of the attendees were seasoned health professionals and policy makers who weren't about to be intimidated by a Bush administration political appointee.

Thompson's method of fielding questions was especially revealing. If things got too close for comfort, he would cut the questioner off in a dismissive and patronizing manner. For example, in response to a question regarding how agricultural policy is undermining public health, Thompson retorted: "I am a farmer. I am not going to criticize my profession." When Mark Fenton (host of PBS's *America's Walking*) asked about increasing federal dollars for public walking and biking paths, Thompson was likewise evasive: "That's Congress. That's not my department—that's transportation," as if it were some sort of separation of powers problem. Then, without missing a beat, he went on to extol his work on this very issue while governor of Wisconsin.[17]

Finally, in the question that would become my motivation for writing this book (as I mentioned earlier), State Representative Charlie Brown, chairman of Indiana's Public Health Committee, asked why, if Coca-Cola was such a responsible corporate citizen, it had sent a team of five lobbyists to kill his school nutrition bill? Thompson became flustered and annoyed, saying he didn't know anything about that. As I sat there watching this sorry display by our nation's top public health official, I wondered why he had agreed to take questions in the first place.

Out-Thompsoning Thompson

In addition to HHS Secretary Thompson, U.S. surgeon general Richard Carmona used the *Time*/ABC Summit on Obesity as an occasion to sing industry's praises. Carmona chaired a panel that consisted of four industry representatives: Niels Christensen, Nestlé; Betsy Holden, Kraft Foods; Shelly Rosen, McDonald's; and Don Short, Coca-Cola. When Carmona started by thanking the panelists for their bold displays of leadership on obesity and underscored the need for all parties to work together on the issue, I knew it would be all downhill from there.

To say that Carmona lobbed the panelists softball questions doesn't come close to describing what happened next. Carmona asked, "What is the responsibility of corporate America in addressing this obesity epidemic?" Nestlé's Christensen said his company anticipates more profit: "We see this as a business opportunity, to develop new value-added products." Holden of Kraft chimed in with: "It's part of our responsibility to be part of the solution." Rosen, the McDonald's representative, took the cake with: "Corporate citizenship is part of our DNA."[18]

Next, Carmona won the prize for the question most guaranteed to get a preprogrammed response: "Do we need lawsuits? Are lawsuits necessary to force corporate America to do their job?" And how did the potential targets of litigation answer? McDonald's Rosen had her predictable rejoinder at the ready: "The answer is clearly no. We believe the way to change behavior needs to be positive and collaborative and to work together with the right solutions."[19]

Kraft's Holden, to no one's surprise, agreed: "I don't think nutrition policies should be decided in a courtroom; often we look for silver bullets when this is a very complex issue and there isn't one sector or industry that's fully to blame."[20] (At this point I started wondering if these answers had been scripted in advance.)

Carmona seemed quite pleased: "I appreciate the comment about the silver bullet, because Americans want instant gratification. But it's taken us decades to get here and I think we have to step back and really deal with this thing realistically to understand that it is going to take quite a long time to change the culture of an entire country."[21] A long time, indeed, especially with government officials fawning all over the very corporations that are a major cause of the problem.

After only a few questions, Carmona wrapped up with the following: "We really need to continue to move forward with this, but rather than creating adversarial situations, my approach is to try and keep all the stakeholders at the table, but keep their feet to the fire, and continue to make those changes that will result in a healthier America."[22] How, exactly, the surgeon general (whose office has no enforcement power to do anything, anyway) was planning to hold industry's "feet to the fire" remains a mystery to this day.

When it became clear that there wasn't enough time for questions from the audience, the tension in the room was palpable as other participants expressed frustration that their voices could not be heard and that, as a result, industry's posturing was left unchallenged.

In the end, I was disappointed that two of the nation's leading media outlets (ABC News and *Time* magazine, who organized the event) would orchestrate such a shameless PR opportunity for leading food companies. What was the point, exactly, of an all-industry panel with no opposing viewpoints and a "moderator" who asked no challenging questions?

Rack Up Another PR Coup for Big Food

One of the sorriest and most depressing events I attended in my entire ten years of covering nutrition policy debates was in July 2005 when the Federal Trade Commission (FTC) and HHS cosponsored a workshop called "Marketing, Self-Regulation, and Childhood Obesity." You might think that when the federal government convenes a meeting on how companies market food to kids, talk of how to regulate industry practices might actually be on the agenda. But you'd be wrong. The whole affair was just another illustration of how government props up industry interests by giving them coveted slots at prominent public meetings.

For starters, from the chairman of the FTC on down, nearly every government official who had the chance made clear that regulation of junk food ads aimed at children was not on the table and wouldn't be anytime soon. FTC Commissioner Thomas Leary went so far as to warn against the government becoming a "nanny state." If this sounds familiar, it's because that's usually the industry's line.

What should have been a serious forum on how to set

limits around the marketing of junk food to children turned into yet another fabulous PR opportunity for Big Food. And no wonder. By conservative estimates, a full two-thirds of the panelists—hand-picked by the FTC and HHS—had financial ties to either the food or advertising industries.

Workshop panelists included representatives from food companies such as General Mills and McDonald's; media companies like Nickelodeon; and advertising agencies catering to food-industry clients. Two powerful trade groups whose mission is to advance the interests of the food industry—the GMA and the Association of National Advertisers—were also invited presenters.

To add insult to injury, executives from Kraft and PepsiCo were each given two separate opportunities to speak, an honor not bestowed on anyone else. The deck could hardly have been stacked any higher. The few voices of public health advocates that did get heard were essentially drowned out by industry.

Moreover, questions from the audience were subject to tight prescreening by panel moderators. Only in response to pressure from advocates did the FTC alter the agenda at the last minute to include a brief "open forum" at the very end of the day, after all the reporters and most attendees had already left. (This was my only opportunity to speak, for a brief few minutes, to the few stragglers still left in the audience.)

Clearly, the government was not interested in hearing from the public on this matter. The main effect of the panels being so biased was that instead of the meeting being about how junk food ads aimed at children should be curtailed, the event turned into a forum for companies to talk about how great a job they are doing promoting "healthier" foods to kids. Indeed, the entire first day was wasted with such posturing.

And the industry should thank the taxpayer for providing it with a very expensive press conference. Among the 350 attendees were reporters from all the major outlets, including the *New York Times*, the *Wall Street Journal*, and the *Washington Post*.

Susan Linn, author of *Consuming Kids*, was one of the few outspoken experts invited to appear. Her panel consisted of representatives from Kraft Foods, PepsiCo, the GMA, and the Association of National Advertisers.

She said the problem wasn't just that her panel was weighted heavily toward industry, but that the whole meeting was. "I was struck by the government's complicity in the food industry's deceit around food marketing to children. No one even suggested that the food industry cut back on marketing junk food. It was disturbing to see that agencies such as the FTC, who should be protecting the public interest, aren't interested in doing their job," she said.[23]

The President's Council on Food-Industry Fitness

The cozy connection between the federal government and industry is further cemented in so-called public-private partnerships aimed at allowing the two sectors to "work together" toward solutions to obesity.

Case in point: the President's Council on Physical Fitness and Sports. Dating back to the Eisenhower administration, the President's Council is an expert committee of volunteer citizens that advises the president through the secretary of health and human services about physical activity, fitness, and sports in the United States. As I said before, I have nothing against physical fitness; it is a critical component of good health. However, the council's focus on this single issue while partnering with major food companies detracts from nutrition policy and other thorny political questions that could spell trouble for industry.

For example, what is a fitness council doing partnering with General Mills, makers of such empty-calorie products as Lucky Charms cereal, Pillsbury cookies, and Häagen Dazs ice cream? Of course, the General Mills Web site speaks glowingly of the partnership:

> In addition to community grants, the General Mills Foundation sponsors up to 50,000 young people to participate in the President's Challenge and earn the Presidential Active Lifestyle Award for their commitment to a physically active and fit lifestyle. Each year, the foundation awards 50 grants of $10,000 each to community-based groups that develop creative ways to help youth adopt a balanced diet and physically active lifestyle.[24]

Sounds impressive, until you realize that the program costs the food giant only $500,000 a year while, in contrast, General Mills reported net sales of $3.27 billion during a *thirteen-week period* in 2005.[25]

Recognizing a good bandwagon when they see one, Burger King, Coca-Cola, and Pepsi-Cola have also entered into partnerships with the President's Challenge.[26] Other examples of public-private partnerships include America on the Move and Shaping America's Youth. (See Appendix 2.)

What's wrong with public-private partnerships? Isn't it a good thing if corporations want to "give back" some of their enormous wealth? Couldn't these good community programs use the money? Of course, but we must also ask what price we are paying. What is the trade-off when government enters into these agreements? What exactly is industry "buying" with its tax-deductible donation?

Getting the government seal of approval is worth a lot to image-conscious companies. They can maximize the halo effect by associating closely with an institution that represents consumer interests (or at least is supposed to). The potential value that food companies gain from this benefit is worth much more than the pittance they paid.

Also, food companies are desperate to ensure that government does not regulate them or criticize their business practices. What better way to accomplish both those goals than to form "partnerships" with Uncle Sam and community-based groups? If the President's Council partners with Burger King, how likely is it that anybody in the president's administration is going to speak out against how the fast-food chain lures children with *Star Wars* toys and other kid-friendly promotions to get them to eat Whoppers and fries? With these arrangements, food companies are essentially buying the government's silence.

Signs that Government is Promoting Food-Industry Interests

Sometimes it's not so easy to tell when federal government

officials are towing the corporate line. Here are some ways to spot what's going on.

Invoking corporate-speak

Government adoption of corporate-speak is one of the more common examples of complicity. If you hear phrases such as *personal responsibility* or *energy balance* coming out of a federal official's mouth, it's a bad sign. Other examples include health promotion messages that focus on weight loss and exercise when the topic at hand is supposed to be nutrition and eating.

Another phrase government uses that comes right out of industry's playbook is *sound science*, as in, "We need sound science before regulating marketing to children." According to industry (and by extension the federal government), any science that goes against corporate financial interests is by definition not sound. This strategy ensures government gridlock for the foreseeable future since plans to attain the allegedly lacking sound science are curiously never made.

Vague nutrition education messages

As we saw with the USDA dietary guidelines, government refuses to give the public clear nutrition messages out of fear of corporate backlash. As Marion Nestle so eloquently explained in *Food Politics*, you will almost never see government messages telling us to eat *less* of anything. Nutrition advice has been rendered completely ineffectual when you see phrases such as: "Get the most nutrition out of your calories," "Find your balance between food and physical activity," and (my personal favorite), "Make smart choices from every food group." You can find all of these sanitized helpful hints and more industry-friendly nutrition advice on the federal government's "MyPyramid" Web site (www.mypyramid.gov).

Corporate executives dominating meetings

Giving major companies a public platform for their self-serving views is a particularly pernicious way in which government furthers corporate interests. When you see a government meeting agenda stacked with food-company executives, it's a sure sign that nothing of substance will be accomplished, and worse, that the meeting has been hijacked and turned into a PR opportunity for industry. Having personally attended or otherwise covered many of these meetings, I now have a list of "usual suspects" who seem to show up every time. (While it can become wearying to sit through the same cheerleading PowerPoint presentations, the upside is that I've learned to decipher a dizzying array of corporate-speak.) The list includes: McDonald's, Coca-Cola, PepsiCo, General Mills, and Kraft Foods. Of course, these companies are eager to take advantage of any PR opportunity Uncle Sam has to offer. I cannot say if other companies turn down government requests to appear, but I suspect that a company like Burger King might not be so willing, since they haven't made as much noise about changing their ways.

Of course, the corollary to corporate dominance of government meetings is the lack of public interest representation. Another sure sign of trouble is when industry critics are conspicuously absent as panelists or government has invited one or two token public health advocates. Another way that government covers its tracks is to invite academic experts to participate. But you have to do your homework to find out how many of these seemingly objective authorities have a history of working for industry, have taken corporate research money, or otherwise demonstrate a pro-industry bias. These days finding such evidence is very easy. For example, for the FTC/HHS meeting agenda on marketing to children, it probably took me less than an hour of Internet research to discover that two-thirds of the panelists had industry ties; this figure included a mix of corporate executives, consultants, and academic experts.

Meeting agenda focused on happy talk

Another sure sign of industry co-optation of a government meeting is when the agenda is full of anything other than ways to regulate food-company practices. While it may seem counterintuitive that government would bother to hold meetings about anything other than actual policymaking, it does happen. For example, panel titles at the FTC/HHS meeting included such red flags as "Current Industry Efforts to Market Foods to Improve Children's Health" and "Current Media Efforts to Foster Healthier Choices for Children," while notably absent were panels that addressed the actual *problem* of junk food marketing to kids, let alone how government could enact regulations.

Industry praising government programs

When industry comes out in support of a government policy (such as an educational program or the latest update of nutrition advice), this spells trouble immediately. A well-timed industry endorsement of Uncle Sam could indicate several things: (1) the policy was heavily influenced by corporate lobbyists, (2) the program was lame from the start, (3) industry is a direct partner in the scheme, or (4) some combination of the above. Whatever the reason, corporate praise for government action is a really bad sign that should immediately raise doubts that anything of value will result.

What's Wrong with This Picture?

When the federal government is complicit with corporations, it becomes increasingly difficult to distinguish between public and private interests. The government speaks with much more authority than food companies do. That's why it's one thing for an industry lobbyist to prattle on about personal responsibility, but when the nation's top health official invokes such rhetoric, the message is much more ominous. That's when government has essentially abdicated its responsibility to protect its citizens.

The federal government's health education programs maintain the focus on the politically safe arena of individual responsibility. But this emphasis detracts from any meaningful debate on nutrition policy, which, of course, keeps the food industry very happy. As long as the "solution" to the nation's diet-related health woes emphasizes individual behavior and not corporate responsibility, all is well in junk food sales.

Finally, when government gives corporations public platforms and forms partnerships with them, this conveniently places industry right where it wants to be: in the position of telling the federal government how to make policy while getting the stamp of approval from agency officials for appearing genuine about solving the problem, ensuring unfettered continuation of the status quo.

I've discussed several ways that government furthers corporate interests, but these examples are by no means exhaustive. There are countless government policies that undermine nutrition and public health in ways that are less obvious. How excessive tax subsidies of corn production result in the ubiquitous sweetener high fructose corn syrup (which some experts say contributes to weight gain) is an excellent illustration.

But I am especially outraged by the examples in this chapter because they are blatant and deliberate strategies to place corporate profits above public interest. It's as if government officials aren't even trying to hide how deeply inside industry's pockets they have buried themselves. It's bad enough to have government do *nothing* when it comes to trying to solve the mess we're in, but when officials go from inaction to *helping further* corporate interests, that's crossing a line that we cannot and should not tolerate. Ultimately, Americans pay the high cost of government complicity—with their health.

8

Co-opting the Science

Line them up and get them on retainer before others do.[1]
—Attorney Carol Hogan, advising food companies
to waste no time in hiring scientific experts

When most people think of the American Diabetes Association, they probably imagine researchers toiling away in the lab in search of a cure, or health educators helping patients. What if I told you that the group is linking arms with Cadbury Schweppes, maker of sugar-filled Dr Pepper and chocolate Creme Egg candy? You'd probably think it was a bad joke, right? But it's deadly serious. Even more disturbing, this partnership is but one indicator of how low America's leading health organizations and professionals are prepared to stoop in exchange for a hefty cash payout from Big Food.

While research has a critical role to play in the ongoing

policy debate around food and health, increasingly, nutrition science is being co-opted by the powerful forces that stand to benefit most from obfuscation of the truth.

The Best Science Industry Can Buy

Food makers like to enlist the services of "third-party," or "nonaffiliated," consultants who specialize in massaging scientific data in industry-friendly directions. I had a rare opportunity to gain an insider perspective on this time-honored corporate strategy straight from the mouth of a hired gun himself. I managed to attend a 2004 gathering of food industry defense counsel called "Legal and Strategic Guide to Minimizing Liability for Obesity: What Food Industry Counsel Need to Know Now." Making no attempt to conceal my identity or background, I struck up a conversation with one Terrence Gaffney, vice president of "product defense" at the Weinberg Group, a scientific consulting firm. (He apparently was not familiar with me or my work.) I asked Gaffney if Weinberg was getting more obesity-related business and he said yes, referencing a client (which he did not identify) from the beverage industry that was especially concerned about the issue of soda and children.

Gaffney enthusiastically explained to me how the Weinberg Group "gathers the science" to support the positions of its food-industry patrons. He boasted that his consulting group itself employs "third-party experts." This is great, he said, because these professionals "have no connection" to either Weinberg or the client company. What's more, they can be used in a number of effective ways. They can give testimony in support of legislation, appear on TV, or write

op-ed articles, for instance—all in support of industry interests.[2] I walked away from the encounter not surprised to
learn this was going on, but still deeply disturbed by
Gaffney's lack of even the faintest hint of ethical qualms.
Quite the opposite; he seemed rather tickled at the under-
handedness of the technique.

Industry wolves in scientists' clothing

To spin the scientific discourse in its favor, the food industry
exploits the third-party approach in numerous ways. One particularly nefarious maneuver is to pay researchers to produce
industry-friendly findings for publication in prestigious academic journals—which sometimes neglect to make those
biases known. A good example is an article titled, "Soft
Drinks, Childhood Overweight and the Role of Nutrition
Educators: Let's Base Our Solutions on Reality and Sound
Science," which appeared in the September 2004 issue of the
Journal of Nutrition Education and Behavior (*JNEB*—a peer-
reviewed "official journal" of the Society for Nutrition Education). It was authored by Liz Marr, a dietitian and partner
in the consulting firm Marr Barr Communications. Marr
Barr's clients include, coincidentally enough, Coca-Cola, the
very same company that funded her work. To its credit, *JNEB*
did reveal this fact to its readers.

However, this disclosure did little to deter Coke from
using Marr's bought-and-paid-for conclusions to defend its
products and practices from critics. For example, the *JNEB*
article was on display at the company's annual shareholder
meeting in April 2005, where Coke was bracing itself for a
public scolding. Moreover, during the session, Coca-Cola

CEO E. Neville Isdell referred to the article by way of defending the firm's marketing practices without bothering to mention that his own company had funded the article.[3] Isdell was especially eager to play up Marr's attempt to dismiss the "myth" that "soft drink companies market to young children." In her article, Marr insisted that "for nearly fifty years, the Coca-Cola Company has adhered to a policy not to market soft drinks to children under the age of twelve years. Recently, the company expanded that policy to apply to all of its beverages, including juices, sports drinks, and water."[4]

But other experts aren't convinced. Josh Golin of the Campaign for a Commercial-Free Childhood attended the shareholder meeting and was appalled by Coke's positioning of the journal article as a PR tool. In a letter to *JNEB*'s editors, Golin noted that Marr was wrong on her facts, citing numerous examples of how Coca-Cola markets to children under age twelve, including product placement on television shows and branded checkers sets. He also questioned the journal's complicity in bolstering Coke's position:

> In short, to dispel the "myth" that soft drink companies market to young children, Marr merely parrots Coca-Cola's false claims about its own marketing practices. But when Coca-Cola makes these claims, some people, at least, may recognize that these are the self-serving words of a company desperately trying to maintain its access to children. When Marr repeats Coke's lies, she speaks with the authority of both her own expertise and the prestigious *Journal of Nutrition Education and Behavior*.[5]

In another example of industry-sponsored research resulting in pro-corporate results, soft drink companies collectively funded a 2004 study to show that soda intake was not linked to decreased calcium. Many health experts are concerned that soda is displacing milk in children's diets. So to counter this negative PR, the American Beverage Association funded research at the Center for Food and Nutrition Policy (CFNP) at Virginia Tech (an institution that regularly accepts corporate largesse). These results were published in the *Journal of the American College of Nutrition*, a peer-reviewed and respected academic publication.

Maureen Storey, PhD, director of CFNP and lead author of the study (and a frequent mouthpiece for the soft drink industry) countered the widely accepted scientific viewpoint that teens are drinking too much soda: "Many people have the mistaken impression that adolescent girls are drinking inordinate amounts of soft drinks," Storey said. "However, it is wrong to suggest that girls are consuming gallons of soda pop when the amount they are drinking, about one can a day, is not excessive if they are physically active."[6]

First of all, these statistics are deceptive. There is plenty of other data to indicate that many teens are in fact drinking more soda than one can a day.[7] In any event, most teens are *not* in fact physically active, so even if we accept Storey's data, her solution, which is to get kids to exercise more, rings hollow. That a respected academic journal perpetuated such corporate spin is shameful.

The corporate takeover of academic research is a growing problem that threatens to undermine the entire scientific process.[8] This danger is particularly worrisome in the case of food and nutrition, given the massive confusion that already pervades the public discourse. A critical corporate strategy is to create confusion and doubt about sound science on food and health. We can thank the popular media for fueling this bewilderment by regularly emphasizing how scientists keep "changing their minds" on nutrition research. The last thing we need is for academic journals to perpetuate this perception.

Front group science—neutral, objective, and heavily bankrolled

In addition to hiring individual consultants and buying published research, pooling their resources and forming scientific front groups is another way food corporations deploy third-party experts. When a Coca-Cola lobbyist shows up to testify against a nutrition bill, the bias is obvious. But Coke's "partiality problem" is minimized when it enlists an apparently independent, "objective" group to do its dirty work. Sometimes representatives will cop to their industry backing, but sometimes not.

When it comes to putting a pro-industry gloss on scientific findings related to diet and health, the industry front group the Center for Consumer Freedom (CCF) is king of the PR empire. And the number-one issue on its junk science hit list is obesity. There is a notable split within the food industry on the question of whether or not to dispute obesity science directly. Most food companies have shied away from explicitly disavowing the existence of an obesity epidemic (probably out of an awareness of how the denial tack backfired on Big Tobacco). Instead, some have formed advisory bodies to "study" the matter. Food manufacturers are leaving the task of dismissing the obesity issue altogether to trade associations and front groups like CCF.

To rebut scientific claims showing a link between obesity and junk food consumption, and establish itself as a respected authority on the issue, CCF has adopted a multi-pronged approach, including: (1) lobbying against nutrition legislation unfriendly to industry interests, (2) preparing well-timed press releases, (3) publishing op-ed articles and letters to the editor, and (4) advertising its views in print and electronic media.

These efforts appear to have borne fruit: despite possessing no identifiable credentials as a scientific body, CCF is now regularly consulted by journalists for its "scientific" insights on public health issues. To make matters worse, the press—always anxious to inject "balance" and a healthy dose of controversy into its reporting—will often position CCF's biased claims as the "other side" of relatively uncontroversial issues. A September 2005 article in the *Los Angeles Times*, for example, drew attention to the increasing prevalence of obesity in the United States and quoted several health experts who explained the data's troubling implications. But instead of leaving it there, the *Times* correspondent found it necessary to create controversy:

Although many experts agree that more children are overweight, there is debate over the reasons and the best ways to tackle the problem. Dan Mindus, a senior analyst at the Center for Consumer Freedom in Washington, said he had no quarrel with the report's findings, but he cited other recent studies that show tremendous drops in the level of children's physical activity and no evidence of higher caloric intake. "Kids aren't running around outside with their friends like they used to. They're spending all their time with computer games and on the Internet," he said. He acknowledged that his group receives some funding from food and beverage companies, but said the organization is nonprofit, nonpartisan, and independent. "In case after case, we see evidence kids aren't eating any more than they used to, but exercising less," he said. "It's almost too easy to blame snacks in school when it's more difficult to try to get kids moving again."[9]

In this piece, the real experts—who would doubtless agree that kids are less active these days, but nevertheless have a broader perspective on the issue—were not even given a chance to rebuke Mindus's alleged scientific views. That a major newspaper like the *Los Angeles Times* would allow CCF's industry-biased statements to go largely unchallenged is remarkable, but by no means unprecedented; such breaches of basic journalistic principles are routinely committed by other media outlets. Curiously, though, in contrast, reporters covering illnesses like AIDS, leukemia, and Lyme disease rarely solicit "opposing" views of "authorities" who deny that these are serious public health concerns. Of course, unlike CCF's Mindus, any such "denial" advocates are not backed by corporate interests working to establish them as credible experts.

Not content to simply allow compliant reporters to do its bidding, CCF also likes to publish well-timed, strategically placed op-ed articles in leading newspapers. Such pieces are likewise aimed at putting an industry-friendly spin on potentially damning scientific studies—while heading off calls for regulatory controls. For example, on August 26, 2004, the *Atlanta Journal-Constitution* (Coca-Cola's hometown paper and a venue that is consistently friendly to CCF's rants) printed an article by the group's director, Rick Berman, titled, "Soft Drink Hysteria Hard to Swallow." In it, Berman trashed a study published that week in the widely respected *Journal of the American Medical Association* (*JAMA*), which showed a clear connection between soda consumption and diabetes. Berman opined, with rhetorical panache: "Frankly, the contortions that the authors went through to demonize soda would make our own gold medal gymnasts proud."[10] Both Berman and the *Journal-Constitution* failed to explain, however, why CCF's corporate-funded posturing should be accepted as more scientifically compelling than *JAMA*'s peer-reviewed research.

CCF is also adept at inserting its pro-industry viewpoints into the popular media the old-fashioned way—through paid advertising. So on April 20, 2005, when the U.S. Centers for Disease Control and Prevention (CDC) announced it was lowering its estimate of annual obesity-related deaths from 365,000 to 112,000, CCF wasted no time getting its PR machine into high gear. A mere five days later, the organization launched a $600,000 media blitz—which included full-page ads in the *New York Times*, *Los Angeles Times*, *Washington Post*, and *USA Today*. In huge letters, the ads dismissed obesity as mere "hype."

CCF's press releases, op-ed articles, letters to the editor, and purchased ad campaigns are shrewd PR tools that are highly effective at sowing doubt about the seriousness of the obesity epidemic, and lending credence to the industry view that its products can be safely consumed as directed.

Second only to the CCF, the American Council on Fitness and Nutrition (ACFN) is one of the most infamous front groups in the business. The name certainly sounds innocuous enough. Who could be against fitness and nutrition? Indeed, according to its Web site, the organization was established with only the noblest of intentions: "ACFN was formed in January 2003 by a coalition of food and beverage companies, trade associations, and nutrition advocates to work toward comprehensive and achievable solutions to the nation's obesity epidemic."[11] Upon closer inspection, however, the group's ulterior motives become clear. Its membership roster includes only a smattering of health groups, but boasts a virtual Who's Who of food-industry trade groups, advertising associations, and top food corporations. (See table for a list of the key industry players on ACFN's executive board alone.[12])

Pursuant to its pro-industry agenda, ACFN has testified before Congress several times on obesity-related matters, doing its best to make sure that the federal government doesn't meddle in the affairs of food makers. Leading the charge on this front is ACFN's main spokesperson, Dr. Susan Finn. Finn's impressive pedigree includes an earlier stint as president of the American Dietetic Association. (The ADA is also a member of ACFN, which should dispel any illusions you might have about the former group's integrity.) Speaking from behind the cover of a seemingly bona fide health organization, Finn is well positioned to dazzle lawmakers with ostensibly authoritative and trustworthy claims about obesity and the futility of government intervention.

In addition to bearing witness before Congress, Finn has written opinion pieces for a number of major newspapers. In November 2003, she penned two letters to the editor—one published in the *Chicago Sun-Times* and the other in the

Oregonian—that neatly encapsulate ACFN's basic position on obesity. In her *Sun-Times* missive, Finn extolled the virtues of individual responsibility and education. "Research," she stressed, "consistently demonstrates that people recognize that they are ultimately responsible for maintaining a healthy weight."[13] Responsibility for the obesity epidemic is thereby shifted away from junk food makers and dumped squarely into the laps of individual consumers.

Disturbingly, both the *Sun-Times* and the *Oregonian* identified Finn only as ACFN's chair, neglecting to reveal her group's industry biases and backing. When media outlets fail to make such corporate affiliations clear, readers are left with the misimpression that writers like Finn are speaking solely from a position of impartial, professional authority.

In reading press reports, it's easy to confuse the American Council on Fitness and Nutrition with the American Council on Science and Health (ACSH), another industry front group with an impressive, neutral-sounding name. ACSH has been shilling for various industries for decades, but has also recently jumped into the obesity fray. ACSH's corporate funders have included Coca-Cola, Burger King, Frito-Lay, General Mills, Kellogg, Kraft, Nestlé, PepsiCo, the American Beverage Association, and the Sugar Association.[14] Like ACFN, ACSH has effectively used the media as a sounding board for its pro-industry ideology. A good example of ACSH's rhetorical handiwork is an editorial by its president, Elizabeth Whelan. Titled "A Year of Public Health Lunacy," the piece appeared in the *New York Post* in December 2005. Topping Whelan's list of "loony" health policies were those pesky grassroots efforts to rid schools of sugary soda:

Public-health advocates have to rally popular sentiment and political support to achieve many of their goals—but increasingly, they seem to put politics before science . . . But banning specific foods won't stop kids from eating other foods, and it's their total calorie intake (vs. calories burned off through exercise) that matters, not a few "evil" foods.[15]

While Whelan tries to masquerade as a bona fide expert, her argument simply reiterates the classic corporate view that everyone knows there are no "good" or "bad" foods. This position nicely jibes with industry's effort to continue to market every unhealthy food product under the sun. It's thus the height of hypocrisy for ACSH to accuse public health advocates of putting politics before science. And it's just as troubling that the *New York Post* (just like the papers that published Finn's opinions) had no compunction about printing Whelan's views without identifying her organization's corporate backing. Be on the lookout for more of ACSH's disguised pro-corporate, science-spinning shenanigans in the future. (For a guide to front groups, see Appendix 2.)

Co-opting the Scientists: Health Advisors for Sale

In addition to outsourcing the science, food makers are increasingly bringing health experts in-house for maximum spin control by inviting them to sit on formal "advisory panels." This tactic burnishes a corporation's reputation by associating it with a body that appears to be "official," "objective," and "impartial." As an added bonus, hiring health professionals often disabuses them of any impulse to speak out critically of industry. As a technique of scientific and academic cooptation, it works like a charm.

Most food-industry leaders have established such advice-giving bodies, including PepsiCo, Kraft, McDonald's, and Coca-Cola. PepsiCo (which owns Frito-Lay, among other major brands) has gone so far as to create a "Blue Ribbon Advisory Board," which includes no fewer than eighteen health experts, eleven of whom are MDs. One of these physicians is the esteemed Dr. David Kessler, former head of the FDA and now dean of the University of California, San Francisco Medical School. Ironically, Kessler is well known for going up against the tobacco industry during his tenure at FDA. What a magnificent coup for PepsiCo, the king of salty snacks, to have netted one of the nation's leading public health figures as an official "consultant."

Also anxious to pursue this path, McDonald's announced the launch of its "Global Advisory Council on Balanced Lifestyles" in May 2003. The fourteen members of this impressive-sounding committee, whose members include former U.S. Health and Human Services director Louis Sullivan, are rewarded with an annual fee of $7,500.[16] Apart from the council, another expert advisor to the fast-food giant is Dean Ornish, an MD best known for promoting a low-fat, mostly vegetarian diet to prevent heart disease. Clearly pleased to have him onboard, McDonald's has dedicated an entire page on its Web site to Ornish's "tips on heart health."[17] Ornish defends his association with the burger chain as "an amazing platform to make a difference"[18]—which also explains why he's embarked on similar partnerships with PepsiCo and ConAgra Foods.

But others are troubled by such cozy relationships between health professionals and large food corporations. Dr. George Blackburn, director of the Center for the Study of Nutrition Medicine at Harvard Medical School, stepped down from McDonald's advisory council in 2005. Blackburn was disappointed that his recommendations on cutting calories and eating quality food "weren't making it through" to the company's Balanced Lifestyles campaign. He complained that the company (not surprisingly) only wanted to promote exercise.[19]

Also determined to create the appearance of being genuinely concerned about health, Kraft Foods has jumped on the consultative committee bandwagon. In September 2003, the conglomerate inaugurated its "Worldwide Health & Wellness Advisory Council," a ten-member panel composed of health professionals from China, Ireland, and Brazil, among other places. The company self-importantly crowed that the body was established as part of its "ongoing commitment to help address the rise in obesity."[20] (When companies really want to show they care, they use heart-tugging words like *commitment*. For more industry-speak, see Appendix 1.)

What's wrong with this picture? For one, forming alliances with top health experts is a pretty good way to ensure that these professionals remain uncritical of your contribution to the nation's diet-related health problems. Similarly, but more importantly, once signed up as "advisors," such experts are extremely unlikely to call for government controls on unsavory corporate practices such as junk food marketing to children. Instead, they're apt to buy into the corporate world's preferred "self-regulatory" approach. With health authorities working hand in glove with them to be "part of the solution," food makers can rest easy in the knowledge that these professionals will obediently refrain from banging on lawmakers' doors to demand pesky, profit-crimping regulations.

If You Can't Beat 'Em, Buy 'Em

Another clever way to control the scientific debate is to establish—with the help of a little cold hard cash—partnerships with professional health associations and disease foundations. By creating such alliances, manufacturers can ensure that these "respectable" groups remain complicit with their take on the relevant science, while scoring valuable PR points.

It's no secret that almost every major health organization from the American Heart Association to the American Cancer Society accepts corporate funding, but it's particularly egregious when certain groups take money from those companies whose products are causing the very problems they are supposedly trying to combat.

In this department, one group has distinguished itself: the American Diabetes Association (ADA), which earns my special Chutzpah Award. To begin with, the ADA boasts a veritable rogue's gallery of corporate funders, including Kraft Foods, J.M. Smucker, General Mills, and H.J. Heinz. If that wasn't bad enough, in April 2005 the organization announced its intention to partner with Cadbury Schweppes. This firm, as mentioned earlier, is famous for its chocolate Creme Egg candy and its soft drink subdivisions, which include 7-Up, Dr Pepper, and Snapple. Described as "a three-year, multimillion-dollar alliance to support the association in its efforts to fight obesity and diabetes in America," the deal means that Cadbury Schweppes will join with the ADA to conduct extensive outreach activities aimed at increasing "consumer awareness of health and wellness, and the importance of making smarter nutritional choices."[21]

Alarmed at the ADA's decision to enter into an unholy alliance with a candy and soda giant, I shared the news with my colleagues at the nonprofit group Commercial Alert (which works to protect children and society at large from the excesses of commercialism), triggering an interesting chain of events. First, Commercial Alert's executive director Gary Ruskin promptly issued a press release that included this pithy observation:

Maybe the American Diabetes Association should rename itself the American Junk Food Association. What will it do for an encore? Start selling candy bars for M&M/Mars? If Cadbury Schweppes really wanted to reduce the incidence of obesity and diabetes, it would stop advertising its high-sugar products, and remove them from our nation's schools. This is just another attempt by a major junk food corporation to obfuscate its responsibility in the epidemic of obesity and diabetes in the United States. The American Diabetes Association should return this corrupt contribution to Cadbury Schweppes immediately.[22]

Next, to get to the bottom of the insanity, the *Corporate Crime Reporter* (*CCR*, a legal newsletter that covers white-collar crime and other corporate malfeasance) approached the ADA directly. The result was a funny but sad interview that revealed both the ignorance and gall of the ADA's chief scientific and medical officer, Dr. Richard Kahn. Kahn claimed, for example, to have never heard of the Center for Science in the Public Interest's well-known report, "Liquid Candy," which describes in detail the myriad public health problems resulting from excess soda consumption. Even worse, Kahn staunchly defended ADA's policy of taking money from companies that contribute to the very health problems his group claims to be working to reduce. Here is a typical exchange from that interview:[23]

Kahn: Most of the companies that give us educational grants are not in the food industry.
CCR: But you do take money even from candy companies.
Kahn: No, I don't think we do take money from candy companies.
CCR: Well, Cadbury Schweppes is a candy company.
Kahn: If we want to prevent diabetes, reduce the prevalence of obesity, help find the cure to diabetes, we have to get funds from someplace.

In another hilarious exchange, Kahn tried to claim that sugar had nothing to do with diabetes:

CCR: There is no evidence that sugar has anything to do with diabetes?

Kahn: None. There is not a shred of evidence that sugar per se has anything to do with getting diabetes.

CCR: Well, weight has something to do with it.

Kahn: Yes, weight has something to do with it.

CCR: Does sugar have something to do with weight?

Kahn: No. Calories has something to do with diabetes.

CCR: Given that sugar has a lot of calories—

Kahn: Anything with calories.

Clearly, forming a partnership with the ADA was an astute move on Cadbury's part. First of all, the deal enabled this leading sugar peddler to buy off the ADA as a potential critic. What's more, by allying with a respected disease foundation, Cadbury gave its corporate image a nice esteem-by-association face-lift. Cadbury even went so far as to pay the ADA for the use of its seal of approval on some of its products. When pressed by CCR, Kahn indicated that this seal would probably be featured only on Cadbury's diet sodas, since they're reduced in calories.[24]

Isn't it nice to know that the ADA has such high nutritional standards? In a follow-up commentary on their interview, corporate watchdogs and *CCR* editors Russell Mokhiber and Robert Weissman noted that the ADA's sellout to Cadbury is part of a larger, and deeply troubling, trend among health associations: "If you are wondering why Americans are losing the wars on cancer, heart disease, and diabetes, you might look at the funding sources of the major public health groups. Big corporations dump big money into these groups."[25]

Truth be told, I haven't had much confidence in the integrity of the major health organizations since attempting to volunteer with my local branch of the American Heart

Association in 1996. Then I was the sole dissenting voice on a conference planning committee and wound up quitting, disgusted that my objections to the group's decision to accept funding from the California Beef Council were not taken seriously. Even so, I find the ADA's involvement with Cadbury even more dispiriting, because of its outright shamelessness—not to mention Richard Kahn's utter cluelessness. By endorsing the products of a soda and candy manufacturer, the ADA is not simply compromising its effectiveness; it's actually contributing to the problem it's charged with addressing. Indeed, if the ADA and other disease foundations have become so desperate for cash that they can no longer see why this sort of corporate funding might be a problem, then maybe it's time for them to close up shop altogether.

Let's Get Together and Form Ourselves an Institute

Another increasingly popular tactic for manipulating and controlling the scientific discourse is to generate industry-friendly "research" under the cover of seemingly impartial institutes founded by food manufacturers themselves. Like corporate advisory panels, such bodies are given lofty, objective-sounding names to convey scientific integrity. Witness the Bell Institute of Health and Nutrition, created by cereal giant General Mills. Its mission is to "contribute to research on whole grains, micronutrients and breakfast, and publish research and scientific articles in leading peer-reviewed journals."[26] The significance of the word "Bell" in the organization's name isn't exactly clear. For me, it conjures up images of pioneering inventor Alexander Graham Bell, slaving away late into the night in pursuit of cutting-edge scientific discoveries and, indeed, the Truth.

Selling science to the highest bidder: the dairy weight-loss scam

General Mills' Bell Institute has generated a number of noteworthy scientific "findings," including the claim that yogurt can contribute to weight loss. Not just any yogurt, of course, but Yoplait yogurt—which just happens to be a General Mills product. A corporate press release proudly explained that participants in an institute-administered study "who included Yoplait Light in their diets also lost 81 percent more fat in the stomach area, which is the most dangerous type of fat."[27] Curiously, neither the press release nor the *International Journal of Obesity* (which published the study even upon peer review) bothered to disclose the fact that General Mills funded the research.

The corporation's Yoplait study was headed by Michael Zemel, PhD, a professor of nutrition at the University of Tennessee. Zemel has accepted nearly $1.7 million in research grants since 1998 from the National Dairy Council.[28] His industry-funded work has formed the basis of a massive $200 million advertising campaign proclaiming the virtues of dairy as a weight-loss aid. He has also taken the unprecedented step of patenting his study results, so that companies must pay him to cite them in their advertisements.[29] In 2005, the Physicians Committee for Responsible Medicine (PCRM) initiated a lawsuit against General Mills, Dannon, and three dairy-industry trade groups, charging them with creating misleading ads based on Zemel's industry-sponsored research. The nonprofit, which also petitioned the federal government to stop the campaigns, says that other researchers have found that dairy products either have no effect on weight or cause weight gain.[30] PCRM had initially included Kraft as a defendant, but dropped the company from the suit after it agreed to end an ad campaign featuring images such as a giant block of cheese engraved with the words BURN MORE FAT. Nevertheless, Kraft's Web site inexplicably continues to tout dairy as a weight-loss aid, appealing to Zemel's studies to corroborate this claim.[31]

Coke's sugar-coated science

Mounting scientific evidence linking America's "liquid candy" obsession to high rates of obesity, coupled with growing controversy over the marketing of soda in schools, have created serious spin-control headaches for Coca-Cola. So in 2004, in an effort to steer the scientific discourse in a more favorable direction, the beverage giant took a page from General Mills and formed its own institute—namely, the Beverage Institute for Health & Wellness. According to Coke's Web site, this newly created body

> is a research organization within the Coca-Cola Company that supports scientific research, education and outreach with a primary focus on beverages. The Institute supports research that increases understanding of the role that beverages can play in diets and health, in developed and developing countries, around the world.[32]

Sounds mighty impressive, doesn't it? And that is precisely the point: to foster the impression that Coke is sincerely committed to helping the impartial scientific discovery process along for the benefit of all humankind. But you don't have to dig too deep beneath this rhetoric to realize that words like "education" and "outreach" are little more than Coke-speak for shameless marketing. The mission's reference to "developing countries" is particularly sinister, given that Coke has recently come under fire for its destructive activities abroad—for example, in India, where it has been accused of contaminating dwindling reserves of drinkable water.[33] Officials estimate that in the state of Rajasthan alone, people in more than fifty villages are facing acute water shortage allegedly due to Coca-Cola operations, and that water levels have dropped up to ten meters since the company started its operations in 2001.[34] Moreover, at 30 million and climbing, India now has the dubious distinction of having more people suffering from diabetes than any other country.[35]

So-called science at soda-sponsored symposia

Since its inception, Coca-Cola's Beverage Institute has funded no fewer than three scholarly conferences related to nutrition and health. In 2005, for example, the Beverage Institute secured the esteemed Harvard Medical School as the forum for a symposium called "The Childhood Obesity Epidemic: Predictors and Strategies for Prevention."[36] There, Dr. Maxime Buyckx, Coca-Cola's "director of nutrition and health sciences" (as oxymoronic as that title sounds) insisted that there is no scientific evidence of a connection between soda consumption and obesity. This despite a Harvard study that concluded that each additional soda a child drinks a day increases her risk of obesity by 60 percent.[37] Buyckx claimed that the study was methodologically flawed and should be treated as merely "hypothesis-generating."[38] Richard Daynard, professor at Northeastern University School of Law and longtime tobacco-control advocate, attended the meeting. He later observed that "Buyckx's statement eerily echoed claims the tobacco companies made about the studies that showed smoking causes lung cancer. They were all just 'hypothesis-generating'!"[39]

Similarly outlandish industry-science yarns were spun at the Coke-sponsored "Managing Sweetness" conference, which was hosted by the Oldways Preservation Trust in Mexico City in November 2004.[40] To ensure maximum media exposure, journalists received free travel and accommodations—a pretty nice perk.[41] Oldways is a self-described "food issues think tank" with a polished image among chefs and other foodies, so it was more than a tad surprising that the group would allow itself to be co-opted by the likes of Coca-Cola.

According to the trade publication *PR Week*, the Oldways "conference aimed to diffuse concerns that sugary foods are a culprit in America's obesity epidemic."[42] The very name of the conference, "Managing Sweetness," was a pretty good indication that sugar would not be criticized for its contribution to America's increasingly expanding waistline. Sure enough, the meeting produced such "bold" scientific "consensus statements" as: "Good health depends on wise management of calories from all food and drink sources, coupled with wise lifestyle choices that include regular exercise."[43]

Oldways is a group that seems to want it both ways. On

the one hand, they have done some laudable work, for example promoting healthful Mediterranean and vegetarian diets. Their Web site notes the importance of "harmonious balances of good nutrition, pleasurable traditional foods, and respect for the earth that could help modern humans live healthier and happier lives,"[44] certainly all worthy goals. And yet in recent years, the organization is turning to corporate sponsorships that run the risk of eroding those values. In addition to the Coke connection, Oldways also partners with the Whole Grains Council, an industry trade group that promotes breads, cereals, cookies, and crackers. As discussed before, the concept of encouraging Americans to eat more whole grains has been widely distorted by purveyors of processed food. The Whole Grains Council Web site, which proudly displays the Oldways partnership, eerily explains that "[f]ast food and industrial food companies are market savvy, and know it is smart to go healthy." That Oldways has no shame in allowing itself to be co-opted by such "savvy" marketers is a disturbing sign of the times.

Shaking the Foundations of Sound Policy-making

Attempting to control the scientific discourse on nutrition and health is a well-honed strategy of the food industry. While this tactic takes numerous forms, its goals are always the same, to: (1) cast doubt on findings that might threaten financial interests; (2) position food makers' own (biased) contributions to the scientific debate as legitimate and authoritative; (3) co-opt experts who would otherwise be critical of business practices; and (4) ensure, ultimately, that people continue to consume food companies' unhealthy products.

In the right hands, science plays a critical role in public policy debates. I certainly don't want to convey the message that we should ignore science; quite the opposite. We need to rely on credible science for sound decision making. That's why it's critical that scientific research remain unfettered by corporate interests. As more and more health experts and organizations slide down the slippery slope of accepting corporate funding, we will ultimately lose a critical tool for effective policymaking.

Ten Tips for Spotting Corporate-backed Science

1. Be on the lookout for pro-industry science disguised as legitimate academic research, even if it's published in a reputable journal. Always try to find out who funded the study or commentary.

2. Be very skeptical of *any* research that is generated directly by corporations. If a claim about a food product sounds too good to be true (e.g., cheese helps you lose weight), it's highly probable that the underlying research is corporate funded.

3. Beware of news articles that attempt to stir up controversy on scientifically uncontroversial issues, such as the connection between soda and obesity.

4. Take quotes from scientific "experts" with no scientific credentials with a liberal grain of salt. "Analysts" from front groups like the CCF are often credited as bona fide research experts in the popular press, despite their lack of qualifications.

5. Don't believe the scientific views of *any* alleged expert

without first verifying in whose name she is conducting research—no matter what high-sounding institution she hails from, be it Harvard, the American Diabetes Association, or Coca-Cola's Beverage Institute. It takes only a few seconds on the Internet to find out if a researcher has a pro-industry bias. When it's not obvious, remain skeptical until you can be sure. Be suspicious of organizations with names like the American Council on Science and Health, which sound overly objective and officious. In fact, the more "impartial" a group's name sounds, the more suspicious I am.

6. The Internet is also a critical tool for researching unfamiliar organizations. While media outlets often reference front groups without identifying their corporate backers, you can sometimes discover the funders by simply clicking the "About Us" tab.

7. When the identities of a front group's funders remain unclear, certain key buzzwords can tip you off. The Coalition for a Healthy and Active America, for instance, is fond of slogans like "commitment to fitness," "freedom to choose," and "responsible and realistic solutions"[45]—phrases taken right out of the food lobby's playbook.

8. Remember that these days, even well-known and highly respected health organizations like the American Diabetes Association are finding it increasingly difficult not to compromise their integrity in exchange for corporate funding. Be wary of their statements and positions. Truly unbiased groups will clearly state that they take no corporate funding.

9. Stay on top of industry efforts to co-opt science and health experts. Professionals and organizations you can trust today may get bought off tomorrow. On the flip side (though it's rare), some authorities do come to realize the error of their ways and remove themselves from the corporate payroll. When in doubt, contact the expert directly for clarification.

9

Eating in the Dark: Nutrition Labeling in Restaurants

Rather than focusing on labeling, we need to focus on education.[1]

—National Restaurant Association

When New York State Assembly member Felix Ortiz proposed that fast-food chains provide basic nutrition information, he became a laughingstock among his own colleagues. The Brooklyn Democrat thought the idea was commonsense—just like the Statewide Child Obesity Education Program law that he steered through Albany, which ensures that nutritionally based education programs are a part of every classroom in New York State. But his proposal this time was treated with sarcasm. One member brought a plate of cookies into the chamber to share with another member, who made light of his own figure: "I did not develop this physique by eating healthy."[2] So why was Ortiz's bill lampooned? The answer lies in understanding the lobbying power of the restaurant industry.

With more and more people eating out these days, nutrition advocates—and politicians like Ortiz—are calling on fast-food and other large chain restaurants to provide information such as calorie count and fat content on menus. While packaged foods sold in retail stores are required to display a "Nutrition Facts" label, restaurants are under no similar legal obligation. Consumer groups such as the Center for Science in the Public Interest (CSPI) have been trying for several years to pass new laws to fill this informational gap. After all, if gas stations have to display octane levels, why not post calories at a fast-food joint? Why should people know more about what goes into their cars than into their own bodies?

True to form, the National Restaurant Association (NRA), whose members include thousands of fast-food franchises and whose customers include untold numbers of power-lunching politicians, has fought the effort tooth and nail. Thus the current Republican-controlled Congress is almost off-limits to activists seeking nutrition labeling, so high has the deck been stacked against them at the federal level. So advocates—including CSPI—have now shifted their focus to state and local legislation. But even here, opposition is fierce. Indeed, none of the thirteen nutrition-labeling bills introduced so far in eleven states and two cities (Washington, D.C. and Philadelphia) has passed. (Eight such bills are pending as of March 2006.) The NRA's lobbying campaign can boast a 100 percent success rate. That's quite a lucky streak.

Why We Need Nutrition Labeling

On a typical day, 130 million Americans eat outside the home, spending $1.4 billion. In a typical year, Americans partake of 70 billion "meal and snack occasions," generating a whopping $511 billion in sales.[3] With that sort of money at stake, it's no wonder restaurants get very nervous when anyone tries to stir the pot.

In 1970, Americans spent just over a quarter of their food dollars outside the home; roughly thirty years later, that figure had jumped to almost half, 48 percent. The average consumer gets one-third of her calories eating out.[4] Data also suggests that over the same period, the average daily calorie intake increased by 24.5 percent, or about 530 calories, and that when eating out, people eat more food, especially higher-calorie food. To make matters worse, this trend appears to be increasing.[5] Another survey showed that nearly all U.S. adults, at one time or other (97 percent), eat at fast-food restaurants.[6] For those of us (like me) who only see the inside of a fast-food joint on long road trips (and even then just to use the restroom), this statistic is a sobering reminder of how the rest of the nation eats.

It's no secret that portion sizes in restaurants are out of control. According to CSPI, it is common for restaurants to serve two to three times more than what is considered a standard serving size. A gander at the gargantuan portions served at many sit-down chains, such as Hardee's "Monster Thickburger" (1,420 calories, 107 grams of fat), gives you the idea. So it should come as no surprise that when we eat out, we consume more calories. Children eat almost twice as many calories in a restaurant meal as when they eat at home.[7]

Most restaurant food is high in what Americans should be eating less of—saturated fat, trans fat, and salt—and low in nutrients. Moreover, restaurants exploit our natural inclination for flavor. According to the NRA, two out of three consumers say that their favorite restaurant foods provide flavor and taste sensations that they cannot easily duplicate in their home kitchens.[8] And no wonder, since many chains use chemical flavoring additives many of us have never heard of, let alone use at home. This is exactly how restaurants hook customers and keep them coming back for more.

Moreover, a study conducted by CSPI found that the calorie content of typical restaurant meals was difficult to measure accurately, even by well-trained nutrition professionals. In fact, the experts' estimates were sometimes off by significant amounts—200 to 600 calories.[9] If even nutrition authorities can't get it right, then consumers are unlikely to do much better.

Nutrition labeling works

One of the happy side effects of nutrition labeling on packaged foods is that it can take a whole lot longer to get the shopping done. If you're one of those people who stands in the aisle comparing product information, you're not alone. One study showed that three-quarters of adults reported using food labels, and another indicated that people who use food labels eat more healthfully. Almost half of the people surveyed reported that the nutrition information on food labels changed their minds about buying a particular product.[10] This, of course, is precisely why the idea of expanding nutrition labeling from packaged food to restaurants has industry shaking in its boots: it works.

The Ultimate Hypocrisy: Education without Information

Corporate resistance to providing nutrition labeling in restaurants offers a particularly good demonstration of industry hypocrisy. In its "talking points," the National Restaurant Association explains that "[r]ather than focusing on labeling, we need to focus on education, the foundation of this issue."[11]

In the debate over the New Jersey bill, Dale Florio, a lobbyist for the New Jersey Restaurant Association, said inexplicably: "People have to take a certain level of responsibility. Increasingly, these types of bills are decreasing people's need to take responsibility."[12]

In order to deflect blame and accountability, many major food companies are fond of claiming that the solution to the nation's obesity epidemic lies in better consumer education and personal responsibility. And yet, industry lobbyists have successfully blocked every attempt to require restaurant chains to post nutrition information in their outlets. How can consumers become more educated or act more responsibly without access to the information they need to make more informed choices? Industry claims they are providing the information to customers in ways other than on menus, but how useful is it really?

While a few large restaurant chains do provide some nutrition information, a recent study found that two-thirds do not.[13] And those that do, tend to offer the information only in a format that's hard to read, outdated, inaccessible, or otherwise not useful. Sometimes menu nutrition information is available only on large wall posters. Ellen Fried, who teaches food law at New York University, recalls stopping at a McDonald's in New York where "they had one of those huge, 'mice type,' nutrition facts posters posted on one wall near the register. However, it was from 1998 or 1999; not sure which, but definitely last century, Arch burger and all. Good for time travelers, but little else."[14]

Another way that chains make it hard to access nutrition information is by relegating it to brochures or company Web sites. Not all chain restaurant goers have access to the Internet, for starters. And among those who do, how many do you think are likely to visit the McDonald's Web site before heading out for a Quarter Pounder and large fries? On-site nutrition booklets are likewise poor vehicles of communication. While, in theory, such pamphlets are available to customers upon request, a Denny's executive admitted at a 2003 hearing on menu labeling that the company's patrons "almost never" ask for brochures, which are generally kept behind the counters and not in plain sight.[15]

Representative Sean Faircloth of Maine contends that nutritional brochures fulfill a specific and strategic purpose: "To create the appearance of accessible information, without the reality of their use. They don't ask you, 'Do you want to supersize that?' in a brochure—they ask you when you are buying the product."[16]

The glaring shortcomings of the current voluntary system of menu labeling have done little to deter the restaurant industry from insisting that it's working just fine. This rosy rhetoric has been roundly criticized by CSPI and other advocates and lawmakers who are calling on restaurants to make nutrition information clearly visible in restaurants at the point of decision-making—on menus and menu boards. Marketers call such positioning "point-of-purchase" and understand that it has the highest impact on consumer behavior, which explains why industry is so dead set against it.

McDonald's Thirty Years of Deception: Déjà Vu All Over Again

Undaunted by such indictments of the self-regulatory approach to menu labeling, McDonald's recently announced its intention to place nutrition information on the "packaging" of most of its menu items. A company press release, opportunely timed to coincide with the media frenzy around the 2006 Winter Olympics, called the move "the latest transparency initiative in the company's thirty-year record of providing nutrition information to help customers make informed choices."[17]

Now that's creative rewriting of history. Let's go back thirty years to when McDonald's fought off a federal proposal to require nutrition labeling on packaging. Ironically, the company used the same arguments that consumer groups now point to as the limitations of this approach.

For example, a 1975 letter from McDonald's to the Food and Drug Administration (FDA) reads: "[Information on packaging] would result in only *post*-purchase communication to the customer. [McDonald's proposed wall mounting] would provide all customers the nutritional information *prior* to consummating a purchase."[18] McDonald's won that battle.

Despite expressing profound distaste for the idea of menu labeling in the 1970s, McDonald's reluctantly agreed to make nutrition information available to its customers a decade later. The about-face was largely the work of reformers like Stephen Gardner, now litigation director for CSPI. In 1986 Gardner worked for the Texas attorney general's office. His office and sister agencies in California and New York persuaded McDonald's and a handful of other major fast-food chains to agree to provide nutrition information through in-restaurant brochures. "We decided," Gardner explains, "that we could make a case that fast-food restaurants were misbranding products because they didn't give people nutrition information; silence is also deceptive."[19] Although Gardner says that the offices of the three attorneys general could have demanded that the companies put nutrition information on every single wrapper, that wasn't feasible because of challenges such as cups being used for several different beverages. Instead, they settled for getting the chains to supply nutrition booklets in every outlet.

Gardner emphasizes that the fast-food sellers' 1980s policy reversal on nutrition labeling was hardly a voluntary act of enlightened goodwill. "It was only under pressure from us they agreed to do it, in exchange for us not suing them," he said. Moreover, of all the companies that Gardner dealt with, McDonald's was the most resistant. Then, when it came time to tell the press, Gardner says, McDonald's jumped the gun. "They put out their own press release the day before we planned to announce our settlement with all of the companies. McDonald's claimed it had decided to give out nutrition information voluntarily, without mentioning that we made them do it," he said.[20]

To add insult to injury, Gardner says that after being compelled to agree to the menu labeling policy, McDonald's had no qualms about seizing it as an opportunity to tout its food as "nutritious." Indeed, in the months following the settlement, the company put out a series of advertisements making precisely such claims. Gardner explains that when his office questioned McDonald's about the ads, it was quick to defend them as accurate. "Nutrition," company executives noted, essentially means "capable of being digested." Gardner explains: "It was McDonald's position that nutrition means it can be consumed and therefore it has nutrition in it; swallow it and it will not kill you. We told them to stop." So how does Gardner react when he hears McDonald's claiming there has been a thirty-year history of providing nutrition information to consumers? "There has been a history of McDonald's and nutrition, yes; but it has not been progress," he said.[21]

History repeated itself once again just a couple of years later—this time foreshadowing the present-day battle. In 1990 McDonald's (along with the rest of the restaurant industry) managed to successfully exempt itself from the Nutrition Labeling and Education Act's updated "Nutrition Facts" law, which required that all packaged foods be labeled with specific nutrition data. While the FDA sought to subject restaurants to the labeling rule as well, President George H. W. Bush's administration bowed to industry pressure.[22] In fact, according to Michael Jacobson, executive director of CSPI (the main consumer group behind the legislation), industry's sway over lawmakers was so great that including restaurants in the labeling regulation would have guaranteed the demise of the entire 1990 bill. Politics by ultimatum works wonders.

Labeling in Today's McDonaldland

If there's one thing I have learned from following the food industry, it's that integrity is usually last on the list of corporate priorities. From McDonald's perspective, the minor skirmishes played out over the past thirty years amount to ancient history. Now, the company has declared its newfound love for the nutrition-labeling concept while claiming that it's been this way all along. However, a few nagging questions remain about McDonald's "bold" new plan to place nutrition information on product packaging.

For example, just how effective is seeing the calories on the wrapper of a cheeseburger you've already purchased? Imagine if, at the grocery store, after buying all your food, along with your change you're handed the "Nutrition Facts" labels from each of the items you just bought.

When asked why the company won't go further and put plain information on menu boards, McDonald's CEO Jim Skinner claimed that it would be too complex and slow down service. Skinner's "complexity" argument is a familiar industry refrain. Here, McDonald's goal is to convince lawmakers and the public at large that industry is taking care of menu-labeling policy on its own, and that government interference would only grind down a system that is working quite smoothly, thank you.

However, as shown time and again throughout this book, the problems plaguing the voluntary approach to food policy reform are myriad. For one, even if we acknowledge that package labeling is marginally useful (better than nothing certainly), how do we know that McDonald's will maintain the policy? Despite their self-congratulatory claims of corporate responsibility, companies such as McDonald's don't act in the interest of consumers, but rather do whatever is politically expedient in that particular moment. Three decades ago, the threat was government-regulated packaged labeling, and McDonald's fought that off successfully. Now that the threat is menu labeling, the company is attempting to deflect attention by providing something far less effective: labels on wrappers, post-purchase.

Showdown in New York

Having grown up in Manhattan, I can attest that New York is dining-out heaven. This might help explain why the food industry donated $4 million to New York State legislative and gubernatorial campaigns between 1999 and 2005.[23] That kind of dough can buy a lot of lobbying clout. And industry expects a good return on its investment, such as fending off meddling do-good politicians.

New York assemblyman Felix Ortiz, whom we met earlier, is one of the most active members of any state legislature when it comes to proposing policies to promote health. Menu labeling in chain restaurants was just one of six bills he introduced in the state's 2004–2005 legislative session to fight obesity and diabetes. Despite meeting with much resistance and ridicule, Ortiz remains undeterred even on his fourth attempt to pass the measure.

The restaurant industry's lobbying strategy is geared to

convincing key legislators to oppose the menu-labeling initia-tive. Lobbying pressure, according to Robert Stern, the pro-gram manager for the New York Assembly's Task Force on Food, Farm and Nutrition Policy, appears to have persuaded at least one New York State assembly member to withdraw her support of Ortiz's bill. In addition to silencing potential backers, industry persuades politicians to actively speak out against the bill.

Restaurant lobbyists attain these goals by intimidating leg-islators with threats of backing opposing candidates in upcoming elections, Ortiz says. This tactic results in law-makers not voting for a bill, even if they think it's the right thing to do. "The restaurant association and others decided to come together to tackle this issue and they spent millions of dollars to kill one particular bill. They have a big lobby and are willing to spend whatever it takes to kill the bill, including putting up opposing candidates. I think they make this clear. Industry is playing games."[24]

Deceit, duplicity, and denial

Robert Stern recalls a discussion he had with the director of the New York restaurant association who claimed that the menu-labeling bill would negatively impact business and result in layoffs, restaurant closures, and so on. (Similar the-sky-is-falling arguments were also made against—ultimately successful—indoor smoking bans.) But the lobbyist went on to insist that Ortiz's nutrition-labeling policy simply wouldn't work because most of the people who eat at chain restaurants wouldn't pay attention or be influenced by it. "Our response," says Stern, "was wait a minute, if people don't care about it, then why are you concerned about the loss of business? If they don't care, they will keep coming to your restaurant, so your argument of loss of business doesn't hold up. We caught them in a contradictory position and said, you can't have it both ways, either people care or they don't care."[25] Stern says that it became clear that industry's lobbyists weren't really interested in trying to negotiate a bill because they always had some other argument. Such argumentation is a common tactic. Whatever line of reasoning is convenient at that particular moment, no matter how contradictory or inconsistent.

Stern notes that Ortiz was even willing to come to a reasonable compromise: he made changes to the bill's language at least twice to accommodate industry concerns. Nevertheless, industry continued to oppose the legislation—claiming it would be too hard to implement. In the end, the restaurant lobby's opposition to the proposed menu-labeling clearly rested on purely philosophical grounds. So, says Stern, there was no longer any point in trying to negotiate further: industry "just didn't like the concept and no matter how much we addressed their concerns, it still didn't matter."[26] Such dealings are par for the course for corporate lobbyists: they will whine about implementation, but when lawmakers act in good faith to try and compromise, they continue to oppose the policy.

Assembly-floor antics

In June 2005, on the last day of the legislative session, Ortiz, after much cajoling, finally convinced powerful New York State Assembly speaker Sheldon Silver to bring his menu-labeling bill to a vote. But the hour was late and law-makers wanted to go home. The debate on the House floor soon degenerated into a protracted and preposterous exercise in futility. Assembly member Daniel O'Donnell (brother of actress/talk show host Rosie and a liberal Democrat) bogged the proceedings down in a bizarre deliberation over the ability of McDonald's workers to consistently salt french fries. O'Donnell was apparently concerned that the data for sodium content might not be accurate. "I've watched the people who work at McDonald's, and they don't measure how much salt they put in their french fries," he said. "So, do you expect that there will be regular training sessions at McDonald's for the saltshaker people to make sure that they're dispensing salt in an appropriate manner?"[27] Laughter ensued. But O'Donnell didn't stop there; he kept haranguing Ortiz over the salty fries and went on to express deep concern over the ability of pizza makers to measure cheese accurately, along with the potential "confusion" caused by twelve-ounce versus fourteen-ounce steaks.

O'Donnell's antics on the assembly floor and his overall hostility to Ortiz's labeling bill helped convince other Democrats to oppose it, joining those Republicans already so inclined. Thus the demise of the measure was effectively ensured, even though a few lawmakers did try to defend it against O'Donnell's grandstanding. Assembly member Richard Gottfried said, "This is not a laughing matter. This is life and death for tens of millions of Americans; it's as simple as that." He explained that the bill was not as complicated as O'Donnell and others were claiming. Then he got to the heart of the matter:

The corporations are going nuts trying to stop this legislation because they know that it may be devastating to some of their sales if the American people actually knew how much poison was in this food. That's what they are afraid of. They're not afraid of getting fined because a kid shakes the saltshaker three times instead of two. They're afraid, as they always are with these things, about the bottom line and whether they are going to lose sales because people are going to walk into their stores and say, "Oh my God! I had no idea there was so much salt and so much fat in the Chicken McNuggets." And that's what the frantic opposition to this bill is all about and that's why this bill is so important.[28]

A refreshing statement of truth at last was spoken. But when the bill was finally called for a vote and it became clear that Ortiz didn't have enough support, he delivered the final word: "I would like to say, with a lot of passion, I withdraw this bill." Ortiz promises to be back again and this time, he says the debate won't be "like the first one, with a bunch of clowns playing around, when this is serious."[29]

While Ortiz's resolve is heartening, it is sad that he has to keep fighting for what should be a slam dunk. What other critical issues are being kept on hold while he comes back for a fourth attempt at this same piece of commonsense legislation? But such details are of no concern to an industry hellbent on undermining the efforts of well-meaning lawmakers state by state.

The Bullying and Double-dealing Spreads Nationwide

The strong-arm tactics of the restaurant lobby are by no means limited to the New York legislature. Another hero in the nutrition wars is Maine Representative Sean Faircloth, who, like Ortiz, has proposed a number of public health measures, only to be stymied by industry. The restaurant lobby has twice killed his bill to require the posting of calories on menu boards in Maine. Faircloth says his legislation has been opposed by the Maine Restaurant Association, the Grocery Manufactures Association (GMA) (representing packaged-food companies nationwide), and a local beverage lobby, even though the latter two groups have no obvious vested interest in the measure. "They are presenting a united front," he explained.[30] Also, given how much soda is sold through restaurants, if people knew how many empty calories are in a large Coke, the result could be decreased beverages sales.

Neither logic nor reasoning need apply

To help mollify industry concerns over cost, Faircloth drafted Maine's menu-labeling legislation to only apply to chains with at least twenty restaurants. He also stressed that such large businesses already reprint their menus as well as customize their menu prices from location to location. "So I kept saying that given the fact that the bill would not require you to change the menus other than your current existing cycle of menu replacement, how can you claim that it will cost more when you already customize menus anyway? They would just ignore me and keep saying how it's going to cost a huge amount. So there is no logic as far as I can tell, that detracts from that reasoning process." Indeed, deflecting attention from the real problem by pointing the finger elsewhere is modus operandi for industry polemicists, says Faircloth: "Whatever the problem is, there's really some other cause, and not the thing we are talking about today."[31]

Another common industry tactic is to trot out a small mom-and-pop restaurant owner to testify and complain about the burden of increased costs. For a restaurant owner with only one or two restaurants, this is a legitimate concern, which is exactly why they are exempt from the bill. But this doesn't seem to stop industry from complaining about a problem that doesn't exist. Representative Faircloth says they don't send in the big chains to testify. "They emphasize local, mom-and-pops, even though the bill wouldn't apply to them—that's the face that's presented to the public and in the media," he said.[32]

Why so much resistance from restaurant chains? "Because they're worried that it will work," Faircloth says. "That people would change their behavior and make some different choices based on the information. And fast-food companies don't like the idea of people having information so they can make informed choices."

The players were different, but the story was jarringly similar, in California in 2004, when industry lobbyists brought down a menu-labeling bill sponsored by state senator Deborah Ortiz. This time it was the industry-backed Center for Consumer Freedom that spearheaded the anti-menu-labeling campaign. Also joining the opposition was the California Restaurant Association, which predictably argued that the proposed law "sent the wrong message about personal choices and responsibility."[33] The bill never even made it out of the Assembly Health Committee. Senator Ortiz lamented to the press how well-meaning politicians were being shot down by industry: "We are being outgunned by the business interests. Even a rational argument now falls on the deaf ears of legislators whose obligations are not to companies but to their constituents."[34]

Next, buy city hall

The general rule of thumb in policymaking is that it's easier to pass pro-consumer measures at the local level. The idea is that you expect less corporate pressure in city government than in state legislatures or Congress. And yet even locally, the same hardball tactics are winning out. Menu-labeling bills introduced in Philadelphia and Washington, D.C. have also failed due to restaurant-industry pressure. The Washington, D.C. bill was brought to the legislature in June 2003 by Council member Phil Mendelson. It was cosponsored by the council chairman along with four other members, meaning that six out of thirteen assembly members backed Mendelson's bill. So what happened?

Mendelson says that the chair of the Health Committee, council member Sandy Allen, was coerced to abandon her support of the bill by the restaurant lobby. "She told me that if I got the votes, she'd move it out of committee, so I worked hard to get the votes. But at the last minute she withdrew the bill, due to industry pressure," he said.[35] As of this writing, Mendelson says the bill is stuck in the Health Committee, which is chaired by council member David Catania, who back in 2003 called the bill "ridiculous." So

Mendelson is not optimistic about the bill's chances. That such a commonsense measure can't even get through such a small legislative body like D.C.'s demonstrates the enormous power and influence of the restaurant lobby.

Calling industry's bluff

For an added twist to industry's hypocritical tendencies, let's look at what happened in Arkansas. As we will see, the National Restaurant Association has been crusading tirelessly to pass state bills that would grant its members protection from obesity-related lawsuits. In February 2005, Arkansas state representative Sam Ledbetter called the industry's bluff. He offered chain restaurants liability protection in exchange for their support of a menu-labeling bill. The idea was that if restaurants are sincere in saying that people should take personal responsibility for their eating behaviors, then they should give people the information they need to make informed decisions. And in exchange, they would get what they say they wanted: protection from an alleged threat of lawsuits.

Yet the restaurant industry was quick to reject Ledbetter's proposal and lobby against the nutrition-labeling bill.[36] A similar deal was stalled in the South Carolina legislature in early 2006. The Hospitality Association of South Carolina explained its opposition by saying it was afraid that doing something so "unique" would place an "undue burden on our restaurants."[37]

What does this tell us? Clearly, it suggests that food corporations fear providing people with information about their products more than the possibility of lawsuits. It also means that industry's argument that the "real solution" to obesity is personal responsibility is just a clever rhetorical smokescreen for its ultimate objective: freedom from regulation.

Independent Shop Outdoes Megabrands

While multinational companies whine about how hard menu labeling is, at least one independent company is proving them wrong. The fast-food restaurant b.good first opened in Boston in 2004 and was so successful that a second location was added in Harvard Square the following year. The concept is traditional fast food made healthy, and the goal is twenty-five locations over seven years. But unlike its larger counterparts, the burgeoning chain is committed to providing customers with nutritional information, even without being forced to do so.

Co-CEO Jon Olinto admits this policy can be a challenge "no matter what kind of restaurant you are" because of all the scientific measurements required, "something that in a hectic kitchen isn't always feasible." Yet, his company ensures the data by hiring nutritionists to analyze the recipes. "As a result, we feel comfortable posting data on our menu board. In fact, it's really important to our concept. We do it because it reinforces our brand. We're all about making fast food 'real'—homemade in a kitchen, not a lab or factory."[38]

Ben Kelley, of the Boston-based Public Health Advocacy Institute, is a regular b.good customer. He calls the company "an excellent exemplar for effectively providing health information for consumers." He also likes that the food is low-cost and tastes good. "This is what they should all be doing," he said.[39]

While Olinto is somewhat sympathetic to McDonald's resistance to menu labeling, he also thinks that it would be easier for the fast-food giant since its products are prepackaged and its operations highly mechanized. He sums up the corporate motivation well: "In the end, their decision reflects that they don't *want* to do it, not that they can't."

How to Fight Back

Countering the restaurant industry's rhetoric is relatively easy once you learn to recognize their arguments. Below are a few examples.

When they say: This bill will force mom-and-pops out of business.

Respond with: Small businesses would not be affected by the legislation since it only applies to chains with at least ten outlets. (In Maine, it was twenty.)

When they say: The requirements would cost too much, even for chains.

Respond with: Many chains already have the information so would not incur any additional costs in analyzing products; the cost of redesigning and updating menus would be modest given the centralization and scope of most chains.

When they say: The policy is too complex because restaurants customize orders too often for the information to be consistently accurate.

Respond with: The legislation only applies to items "as offered for sale" and does not affect customized orders or daily specials; it also allows for variation.

When they say: When people eat out, they want to splurge and don't want to know the nutrition information.
Respond with: Polls show two-thirds of Americans support the idea; they should not be deprived of information because a minority prefers to remain in the dark.

For a more complete list of arguments and responses, see "Myths vs. Reality: Nutrition Labeling at Fast-Food and Other Chain Restaurants," from the Center for Science in the Public Interest, reprinted in appendix 3.

Remaining Part of the Problem

The louder megachain restaurants like McDonald's complain that it can't be done, the more hollow their position becomes. That the restaurant industry is so frightened by the prospect of giving its customers basic nutrition information speaks volumes. One reason that the owners of b.good aren't afraid of sharing information is that they are selling relatively healthy fare. But with most chains promoting anything but, and with increasing public awareness of the health consequences of a steady diet of Big Macs, disclosing how much fat, sugar, and salt is in a typical fast-food meal is potentially very bad for business.

Moreover, restaurant chains are panicked about the encroachment of any government regulation, however slight, since that could open the door to more oversight. This explains why, even when New York Assembly member Felix Ortiz was willing to negotiate, corporate lobbyists balked. Why bother to compromise when killing a bill altogether is so much more effective? Industry's hard-line position goes to the heart of their utter disingenuousness and hypocrisy. If food companies really wanted to be "part of the solution," they would stop obstructing well-meaning lawmakers from passing these commonsense policies. Instead, they are doing everything they can to remain part of the problem.

10

Battling Big Food
in Schools

The school system is where you build brand loyalty.[1]

—John Alm, president and chief operating officer,
Coca-Cola Enterprises

When state senator Deborah Ortiz proposed legislation to rid California schools of soda and other unhealthy drinks, she expected a fight. But she couldn't have predicted that her age and marital status would get dragged into the debate that followed. Considering the numerous other hardball tactics that industry lobbyists are deploying in the battle over school food, this example may seem tame by comparison.

Public health experts and pediatricians have been sounding the alarm in recent years over the rise in childhood obesity and illnesses previously seen only in adults, such as diabetes and early heart disease. Because of these concerns, children and schools deserve a special place in understanding the national debate over food choices and good nutrition. Children spend a good chunk of their waking hours at school, which has the potential to provide a critical opportunity to teach kids about healthy habits that can last a lifetime. Corporations, however, are taking advantage of schools to reach children in a captive environment.

This chapter describes how the food and beverage industries have systematically blocked every effort to regulate the sale of their unhealthy products in schools and how to fight back. This battle is about more than just public health; it's about allowing corporations unfettered access to impressionable children and youth. At stake for industry isn't just the money gained from school sales. Companies like Coca-Cola are desperate to remain in schools for several reasons: (1) to build brand loyalty among a captive and impressionable audience, (2) to further their positive image by promoting the myth of corporate philanthropy, (3) to avoid the potential harm to their products' reputation outside schools.

How Did We Get into This Mess?

While nominal federal nutrition standards do exist for school meals, for all other school food sales, it's a junk food free-for-all that makes your corner mini-mart look like a health food store. Other authors have amply demonstrated how food and beverage companies market their unhealthy products incessantly to children, especially in schools.[2] A 2003 government survey showed that 43 percent of elementary schools, 74 percent of middle schools, and 98 percent of high schools sold food through vending machines, snack bars, or other venues outside the federally supported school meal programs.[3] Such food items are known as "competitive food" because they undermine tax-supported lunches. In spring 2004, a survey by the Center for Science in the Public Interest (CSPI) revealed that 75 percent of beverage options and 85 percent of snacks in school vending machines were of poor nutritional quality.[4]

To understand how we got here, let's go back a few decades. In 1977, concerns over school nutrition led Congress to direct the U.S. Department of Agriculture (USDA) to limit access to junk food and soda in schools. The reasoning was that federal funding for school meals was being undermined by students' easy access to competitive foods. In other words, kids were loading up on soda and snacks for lunch. However, the soda industry filed a lawsuit challenging the USDA rules, and in 1983, a federal court agreed that the agency had overstepped its authority.[5] So despite Congress's clear intent, legal maneuvering by soda companies allowed schools to swing their doors wide open.

With public schools so desperate for funding, districts are lured into signing exclusive contracts (also known as "pouring rights" deals) with major beverage companies—mainly Coca-Cola and PepsiCo. Often these deals are presented as being very lucrative to districts, with schools offered enticing incentives such as sports marquees or cash bonuses to sign. Moreover, soda companies make the deals seem like a charitable donation when the reality is that schools benefit far less than the companies do. Sometimes these contracts can lock a district in for many years with the same vendor and the same unhealthy options. Usually the amount of money a school district receives is dependent on soda sales, thus creating a conflict of interest between health and profit. In addition to soda, schools sell chips, candy, cakes, cookies, you name it. One angry parent sent me a photo of her child's school store that looked like the inside of a candy shop.

Not willing to take it anymore, from Philadelphia to Seattle, from California to Connecticut, parents, teachers, policy makers, and advocates are organizing to take back their schools from the clutches of Coke and Pepsi. But as advocates are learning, megacorporations don't go down without a fight, not with so much money at stake.

From 2003 to 2005, almost every state proposed legislation to address the sale of soda and junk food in public schools. Despite all the activity, results have been mixed. Many state policy makers have heard the rallying cry from nutrition advocates and are doing their best to respond against all odds. But only twenty-one states were successful in passing any bills during that period, and in at least ten instances, the bills were watered down, a result of political lobbying and compromise. In many other states, the bill as introduced was already weak and likely ineffective, another by-product of corporate pressure.

By all accounts, state proposals to rid schools of unhealthy food and beverages enjoy overwhelming public support. So what's going on? Why can't lawmakers get these common-sense bills enacted? While the food industry may not deserve all of the blame for failed state legislation (sometimes even school officials are opposed), in almost all states where bills fail or are weakened, trade associations and individual companies have a heavy hand in the lobbying.

Sending in the Biggest Guns to Lobby and Distort the Truth

Despite its public claims to being part of the solution, at every opportunity, the Grocery Manufacturer's Association (GMA) puts its members' economic interests above children's health. As mentioned before, the GMA's 120 members enjoy annual sales of more than $680 billion in the United States alone, and consist of major packaged-food corporations such as Kraft, Mars, and PepsiCo. It's standard operating procedure for companies to join trade associations to lobby on the members' behalf to maximize efficiency and power. Another advantage, as we have seen in previous chapters, is that trade groups can do the dirty work without tarnishing the individual corporate image.

The GMA is on record as opposing virtually every state bill across the nation that would restrict the sale of junk food or soda in schools. A search for the word "schools" on the GMA Web site resulted in no fewer than 126 hits, most of which are either submitted testimony or a letter filed in opposition to a school-related nutrition policy. Here are just a few examples of document titles: GMA Letter in Opposition of Texas Food and Beverage Restrictions, GMA Letter in Opposition to Oregon School Restrictions Bills, GMA Requests Veto of Kentucky School Restrictions Bill, and GMA Letter in Opposition to California School Nutrition Bill.

GMA does more than just write letters; the group also has resources to send lobbyists to every state capital in the nation to defeat or weaken legislation. This high-powered lobbying campaign is quite effective. For example, in 2004, GMA helped defeat a California bill that would have set nutrition standards on school food. At every step along the way, the

GMA and its member companies have beat nutrition advocates back because they have more lobbying resources, not to mention money to offer politicians in the form of campaign contributions.

In addition to the national trade associations, individual companies have also undermined numerous state efforts. While the GMA appears to represent mainly the food companies' interests, the soda industry is well represented by high-powered lobbyists and regional bottling associations. When it comes to school nutrition, the one company that emerges as the worse corporate actor is Coca-Cola. While other companies also lobby, Coca-Cola puts up the biggest fight and in the nastiest ways. The general rule of thumb that companies like to leave the dirty work to trade groups does not seem to apply to Coke's lobbyists. Here are three case studies that illustrate just some of the underhanded lobbying tactics used by industry, including misrepresenting the science, disingenuous arguments, and personal attacks.

California's Soda Ban and Politics by Ultimatum

Often a policy bellwether for the nation, California has been a hotbed of activity over school nutrition for years. For example, the Los Angeles Unified School District (the nation's second largest) unanimously passed a policy that took effect in 2004 to no longer allow the sale of soda in schools, becoming the first in the nation to do so. In 2003, grassroots momentum resulted in proposed legislation that would have banned soda sales in all public schools throughout the entire state, kindergarten through twelfth grade. The nonprofit advocacy group California Center for Public Health Advocacy (CCPHA) led the charge to pass this groundbreaking bill, which was sponsored by California state senator Deborah Ortiz.

CCPHA and others presented overwhelming scientific evidence of a growing public health menace caused by children drinking too much soda, much of which is consumed at school. What should have been a no-brainer—protecting kids' health—turned into a bitter battle involving industry's heaviest hitters.

Lobbying machine descends on Sacramento

Wasting no time, the soda industry mounted a strong opposition. According to one observer, "You could see the Coke and Pepsi lobbyists running down the halls after the legislators. They were out in full force."[6] According to Senator Ortiz, the industry front group Center for Consumer Freedom (CCF) hired two lobbying firms known for raising money for Republicans and moderate Democrats. Also, a nutritionist representing CCF testified against the bill, but did not disclose her affiliation and bias—a typical industry tactic.

The soda industry also sent paid consultants to testify at hearings on Philadelphia's districtwide policy without revealing their affiliation. These experts presented industry-sponsored data to show that soda does not cause obesity. How can lawmakers trust the testimony of a so-called expert if they don't know who is paying the bills? As explained previously, corporations hire "third-party experts" who have no obvious affiliation with industry. This way, the expert's research credentials serve as the basis for their credibility and the testimony is deemed objective and scientific. Trouble is, bought-and-paid-for science is anything but objective and can easily be manipulated to obtain the desired outcome. The tobacco industry wrote the book on that tactic decades ago.

Also, as we've seen, another typical industry tactic is personal attacks, which come in handy when you can't argue the facts. Senator Ortiz came under attack numerous times by CCF for her nutrition-advocacy efforts. "Their tactics are horrific; their strategy is to attack the individual to discredit them. And this can get very ugly," she said.[7] CCF's verbal assaults against Ortiz even included obscure references to her being forty and single. When I later shared this story with a colleague who studies tobacco-industry tactics (including how they target homosexuals), she explained that this is a subtle way of suggesting that Ortiz is a lesbian. Those crazy Californians—how can you trust them to make sound school nutrition policy if they can't even manage to get married by age forty?

High school kids on the chopping block

A combination of behind-the-scenes and up-front industry lobbying on the soda ban bill resulted in a proposed amendment that would allow high schools to be exempt. Not coincidentally, most sodas in schools are sold at the high school level. Such an exemption was never the intention of either the nutrition advocates or of Senator Ortiz, the people actually proposing the policy in the first place.

Yet what ensued was a legislative debate over whether high school students were "old enough" to make their own choices when it comes to drinking soda. This served as a convenient smokescreen for what was really at stake: the huge economic benefit to industry to maintain their significant presence in high schools. Behind the scenes, industry put pressure on certain key members of the California Assembly to do their bidding.

For example, Dario Frommer, then chair of the Assembly Health Committee and obviously in industry's pocket, made the absurd argument that many high school students were eighteen years old, able to vote, could serve in the military, so should be able to make their own decisions. But Senator Ortiz countered that at most, only twelfth-graders, and for only half their year, are eighteen. "And it's a time at which key decisions are being made, and thus where industry has the greatest marketing advantage," she said.

In the end, corporate lobbying forced an ultimatum. Either Ortiz's bill would die in its entirety, or it would survive—but banning sodas only for kindergarten through eighth grade. Ortiz took the compromise, but was very frustrated: "I was prepared to have the bill die. I really felt it was a compromise that was unacceptable. But the advocates felt it was a win, and I allowed them to make the call. The food and beverage industries are extremely powerful," she said.[8]

But some advocates were also troubled by the weakened legislation, including Jacqueline Domac, who helped get soda and junk food banned throughout the Los Angeles Unified School District. "I find it quite interesting that we only care about kids until the eighth grade and suddenly in high school, their health is insignificant. As a high school teacher, how do I explain to my students they are just not important to lawmakers?" she asks. Why is exempting high schools so critical to industry? Domac says it's all about brand loyalty.

"It's during the high school years that kids form lifestyle habits. That's when a student decides between Coke and Pepsi, and that lasts for a lifetime," she said.[9]

Advocates were successful in 2005 in passing another law to finally get sodas out of California high schools, thanks in part to backing by Republican governor Arnold Schwarzenegger. But even that bill had compromises. For example, sugary "sports drinks" are still allowed. Also, the law permits a long phase-in period, with full compliance not required until 2009. This gives beverage companies plenty of time to potentially regroup and figure out a work-around.

Kentucky's Four-Year Battle with Coca-Cola

After three previously unsuccessful attempts to improve the nutritional content of products in school vending machines in Kentucky, in March 2005, the state legislature finally passed a compromise bill that removed all soda, but only from elementary schools. Veteran dietitian Carolyn Dennis, chair of the Kentucky Action for Healthy Kids Task Force, battled Coca-Cola lobbyists for four years.

Kentucky had already required that vending machines remain turned off until thirty minutes after the last lunch period. However, as is often the case, that rule wasn't enforced, and many schools disregarded it. Dennis says the machines were turned on first thing in the morning. "And these little kids, they have no judgment; they spend all of their money on candy bars, Coke, and potato chips. And that's what they eat for breakfast, and for lunch," she said. Some elementary school principals even were announcing "soft drink breaks" in the afternoon. Dennis explains:

One of my task force members was giving a health talk to third-graders—that's eight- and nine-year-old children. She was interrupted at 2 p.m. when the principal came over the loudspeaker and said, "OK, children, it's time for your afternoon soft drink break," at which point, all but four or five children who couldn't afford it took their money and followed the teacher out the door, and came back with their 20-ounce Coke or Pepsi, and she continued her health talk. She couldn't believe it; no one made any connection.[10]

As a result of these and similar problems, Dennis joined a coalition to pass legislation to set nutrition standards. "The first year," Dennis recalls, "the NSDA [National Soft Drink Association—now the American Beverage Association] sent four lobbyists to kill the bill." The local Kentucky Beverage Association (KBA) representative, Ray Gillespie, testified that "there were no soft drinks in elementary schools," remembers Dennis, "which was totally a lie." A survey of Kentucky schools had revealed that 44 percent of elementary schools had vending machines, despite Coca-Cola's written policy to not sell soda to elementary schools. Yet for three years Coke's lobbying won out.

On the fourth attempt, Coke offered the elementary school compromise. Allowing schools to continue to sell soda in middle and high schools was the only way the bill could possibly pass. According to Dennis, "We tried to get 75 percent of beverages to be healthy K–12, but the beverage association went ballistic on that one because they wanted to be able to sell Gatorade and the rest."[11]

Coca-Cola's lobbyist even objected to using the language

"healthy beverages" to replace soda, apparently worried about the implications for its reputation. Coke said they could live with a ban in elementary schools but only if the bill did not say "healthy." Dennis explains, "The Coke lobbyist wanted the language, 'school-day appropriate beverages.' We debated it for hours, and finally my colleagues said, 'Look, if this will get them off our backs, let's do it.' Then we compromised on 'school-day approved,' which I didn't agree with because I don't like the word 'approved.' " Dennis likens the experience to a David vs. Goliath battle:

> All these lobbyists work together. The Grocery Manufacturers Association fought us big-time, too. I saw them working with the soft drink lobbyists a lot. I was told the very first year by someone from the ethics commission that next to the pharmaceutical association, you are up against the second-biggest lobby going, and that's the soft drink lobby.[12]

Dennis's team also started tracking campaign contributions. "One of our task force members filed an ethics complaint against the president of the state senate because he accepted money from the soft drink industry. We found that a whole lot of legislators accept money from them, it doesn't matter which party or which chamber you're in," she said.

Showdown in Connecticut: Governor's Coke Connections

In June 2005, Connecticut governor Jodi Rell vetoed what would have been the nation's strongest school-based nutrition law. With one stroke of the pen, she put to rest an extremely contentious battle to rid Connecticut schools of soda and junk food. This was the fourth try to get a bill passed in Connecticut. In 2004, advocates attempted to set nutrition guidelines on food and beverages, but ended up with a gutted law thanks to lobbying by Coca-Cola and PepsiCo.

The 2005 bill would have allowed only water, juice, and milk to be sold during the school day, K–12. To do its bidding, Coca-Cola hired Patrick Sullivan, of Sullivan & LeShane, called "the most influential lobbying firm in the state."[13] For his services, Sullivan is paid $80,000 annually by Coca-Cola's New York division, plus an additional $7,350 a month by its New England subsidiary.[14] The Connecticut Pepsi Bottlers Association hired Jay F. Malcynsky of Gaffney, Bennett & Associates, the biggest lobbying firm in Connecticut. According to Ethics Commission records, Pepsi pays Gaffney, Bennett $50,000 a year in fees. Together, the two firms spent a quarter of a million dollars trying to kill the Connecticut bill.[15] With that kind of money getting thrown around, it's no wonder things got ugly. Really ugly.

The political struggle involved an eight-hour House debate in which lawmakers engaged in such absurd stall tactics as relating memories of being deprived of candy as a child. The House finally passed a compromise bill that allowed diet soda and sports drinks to be sold in high schools after the lunch period. Then the bill had to go back to the Senate, where it had already passed. But this time, lawmakers there attempted to delay the process by adding no fewer than ten unrelated amendments, such as requiring smoke detectors in school bathrooms.

Other underhanded tactics included Coca-Cola's lobbyists sharing data regarding school income from soda sales with lawmakers behind closed doors so that advocates could not refute the information. Also, a well-stocked Coca-Cola cooler was delivered to the Democratic caucus room in the capitol just before the House was expected to vote on the bill. Lucy Nolan, executive director of End Hunger Connecticut, the bill's lead sponsor, called the timing "very suspicious."[16]

And in a particularly devious move, while the bill awaited the governor's signature, a sign mysteriously appeared taped to the inside of the glass on the front of a high school vending machine that read: "Let the state know how you feel about the state getting into your lunch program," followed by Governor Rell's e-mail address and phone number. It's unclear who was responsible for this cheap shot.

Lucy Nolan's group lined up an impressive array of supporters, including the American Academy of Pediatrics, the American College of Preventive Medicine, the American Diabetes Association, the American Heart Association, the Connecticut PTA, the Connecticut State Dental Association, and the Connecticut Nurses Association, hardly a bunch of radicals. Also, according to one survey, 70 percent of the state's residents favored the bill.

In the end, even with overwhelming public support, the compromise bill was too much for the governor to sign. Ironically, the most common argument made against such bills is that schools should maintain "local control" over nutrition policy. Indeed, Governor Rell invoked the word "local" no fewer than sixteen times in her three-page veto message. However, her reasoning is hard to swallow. Many school policies are made at the state and even national level, such as President Bush's notorious "No Child Left Behind" policy.

What Governor Rell failed to mention in her veto message was a possible conflict of interest: the cofounder of Coca-Cola's lobbying firm, Patricia LeShane, served as the governor's campaign advisor.[17] Also, the LeShane lobbying firm contributed to Rell's successful 2002 campaign for lieutenant governor.[18] The lobbying money spent fighting this bill was so influential that it motivated the state's Senate President Pro Tem Donald Williams Jr. (a strong proponent of the nutrition bill) to take concerted action for the first time on campaign finance reform.

Postscript: As of this writing, Nolan was back in the state legislature for a fifth time, trying to pass a compromise measure with backing from the governor's office. But what she thought would be an easier fight is actually just more business as usual. In fact, now Coke is on her back: "The soda lobbyists literally stalk me at the capitol. There is not one place I can go without someone following me. Guess I should feel flattered," she said.[19] The compromise bill did finally pass after much political wrangling.

Rinse, Repeat: Same Story All Over the Nation

Together, Coca-Cola, PepsiCo, national and regional soft drink associations, the GMA and other business groups have undermined school nutrition policies with heavy-handed lobbying tactics all over the nation. Here are just a few more examples of policies that were compromised or completely killed as a result of corporate pressure:

Arizona: In April 2005, Arizona passed a law that bans the sale of soft drinks and candy during the school day, but only for grades K–8. High schools were exempted as a compromise due to heavy industry lobbying. The provision that would have extended the ban to high schools was added and removed from the bill several times, and, ultimately, the soda lobby won.

Indiana: As mentioned before, in June 2004, at the Summit on Obesity sponsored by *Time* magazine and ABC News, Tommy Thompson, then U.S. secretary of health and human services, claimed that Coca-Cola was a responsible company. In response, Charlie Brown, chairman of Indiana's Public Health Committee, asked why such a responsible corporate citizen would send a team of five lobbyists (including a regional vice president) to defeat his bill that would have reduced soda sales in schools by just 50 percent.

Louisiana: In 2005, Coca-Cola enlisted the support of principals who had exclusive soda contracts with the company to oppose a strong state bill to get soda out of schools. Coca-Cola lobbyists successfully proposed a "compromise" in which high schools could still sell 50 percent unhealthy snacks and beverages. Dr. Thomas Farley, of Tulane University School of Public Health and Tropical Medicine, thinks this "50 percent solution" will have a minimal effect at best. "In the end, the governor declared victory, but the victory really belongs to Coke."[20]

New Mexico: After a hard-fought battle in 2005 in the state legislature, pediatricians, school food directors and nutritionists gained approval to appoint an expert committee with the authority to establish nutrition standards for schools, with just one catch: the compromise legislation required the committee to include representatives of the beverage and food industry. At the first committee meeting, Danielle Greenburg, a doctor and obesity researcher, said that banning soft drinks in schools isn't the solution; rather, students need to be educated on how to balance what they eat. This doctor works for Pepsi.[21]

Oregon: What started out as a relatively strong piece of state legislation in 2005 was completely gutted thanks to soda industry lobbying. The original bill would have set strict requirements for school beverages and snacks. The bill that passed, however, only required schools to have wellness policies. An Oregon newspaper editorial squarely placed the blame on politicians bowing to corporate pressure. Three key lawmakers each received $2,000 of the total $91,000 the soft drink lobby poured into legislators' coffers.[22]

Washington, D.C.: In 2003, D.C. Public Schools (DCPS) embarked on an effort to improve the beverage options that were supplied by Coca-Cola. But the company engaged in a concerted campaign to stall the effort. Foot-dragging took the form of claiming to conduct feasibility studies and economic analyses as well as never returning phone calls or e-mails. Coca-Cola Enterprises sent a vice president to a meeting with DCPS to challenge the nutrition standards that advocates had put forward, complaining that the company had not been adequately consulted and would lose money.[23]

Washington State: In 2004, the state tried to pass legislation that would have banned selling junk food and soda in schools. But, according to Seattle School Board member Brita Butler-Wall, seventeen revisions later, the bill was watered down significantly: "It's pretty weak. It requires that by the fall of 2005, all schools have some sort of policy around junk food and soda." She suspects Coke had an influence on the outcome: "Just a few days after we sat down with my legislator to talk about this, Coca-Cola sent out a couple of its representatives from Atlanta to meet with her. So that certainly didn't help matters."[24]

So while Coca-Cola and PespiCo are trying to position themselves as "part of the solution" by providing schools with "free" educational materials on nutrition and exercise, behind the scenes, they are undermining school nutrition policy.

Rhetoric and Spin: Countering the Arguments

An important tool in going up against the powerful food and beverage industries is to anticipate their arguments, and then be ready to counter them. Sometimes, reframing the issues can help convince key policy makers. Here are a few of the typical arguments made in the battle over soda and junk food in schools.

Whose choice exactly?

The soda industry is especially fond of evoking all-American values such as "freedom" and "choice." Kari Bjorhus is Coca-Cola's director of "health and nutrition communications" (this must be a fun job). She assured me that the company "offers a wide variety of beverage choices and it's up to the school to decide which beverages they want to offer their students."[25] Indeed, the company has an entire "program" it calls "Your Power to Choose," which it created in response to the school debate. (Never mind that Coke interferes with schools that are *trying* to choose healthier beverages.

By preying on Americans' inherent sense of individualism, industry is twisting the concept of choice. Upon closer inspection, the question becomes: who exactly is making the choices and who benefits financially? You only need to read the language of an exclusive soda contract with a school to understand that the companies call all the shots, making such decisions as what products are sold and how much is sold, even down to the number of ounces. Also, the very nature of an exclusive contract restricts choice because schools cannot bring in healthier beverages from other vendors without risking violating the contract.

The freedom of choice argument was made in the California battle over soda in high schools—that high school students should be able to make their own "choices." But Michael Butler, legislative advocate for the California State PTA, says that's not a valid argument. "I can understand students making healthy choices. But we don't put cigarette vending machines in high schools to allow students to have a 'choice,' " he said.[26] Also, we make all sorts of choices for high school students. The very fact that we even still require them to attend school means that as a society, we are making decisions regarding their well-being that limit their choice—because it's in their best interests.

Maine state representative Sean Faircloth finds the concern over freedom of choice amusing. "Yes, we definitely do have a freedom of choice problem—you can't get the healthy stuff! By improving the options in vending machines, the school would be creating a small island of opportunity for healthy choices. Trust me, as soon as kids leave the school grounds, they will be flooded with corporate advertising. We should start with the premise that schools should not be designed to create branding opportunities," he said.[27]

Exploiting schools?

Another disingenuous and self-serving argument is that schools will suffer if they don't continue to sell children soda and junk food. While it's true that schools are in desperate need of money, we should be asking: is the solution to that problem really getting children to load up on products that make them sick? We shouldn't be trading children's health for after-school programs. Also, evidence is emerging to show that exclusive soda contracts don't actually bring schools as much money as Coke and Pepsi would have us believe. For example, a report from Oregon analyzing soda contracts in that state found total revenues for districts ranged between $12 and $24 per student annually and concluded that contracts are more lucrative for vendors than for school districts.[28]

Let the locals decide

Another common argument against creating a statewide nutrition policy is that schools should have "local control." This justification is made by Coca-Cola's Bjorhus: "A lot of people feel very strongly about local control—for parents and local school administrators to have the flexibility to make decisions that are right for them."[29] But in California, even local control proponents such as the Association of California School Administrators (ACSA) were in support of statewide standards, so on behalf of whom exactly was Coca-Cola arguing?

"Local control is a premium," says Brett McFadden, legislative advocate for the ACSA. He admits that it took some time for his members to come around to supporting statewide guidelines, but they eventually realized that childhood obesity was too important. "When there is a broader statewide interest in establishing policy, then the state has both a responsibility and an obligation to set that policy," he said.[30] Michael Butler agrees, saying that "the California State PTA believes in local control when it serves the best interest of all children and youth, not when it serves to accelerate the sales of carbonated beverages."[31]

Also, what about parental control? Kentucky's Carolyn Dennis says that nothing is more local than her right as a parent. "Schools are interfering with parental control, just to make a profit at the expense at our children's health. You are interfering with my rights as a parent," she said.[32]

It's classic doublespeak for industry to argue local control. Whenever you hear an argument from industry, simply ask yourself, who benefits economically? Obviously, Coke and Pepsi are in no position to argue that schools deserve to have local control over these decisions when the companies are the direct beneficiaries of such a policy. It's laughable to imagine the largest beverage companies in the world arguing on behalf of the poor, treaded-upon school districts supposedly getting beat up by state policy makers who are taking away their rights. Whenever you hear a multinational corporation stand up for the little guy, this should instantly make you suspicious. If Coke and Pepsi were to make more money through "federal control," you'd hear them arguing that the feds should determine school beverage policy. Once you understand how self-serving industry's arguments are, it's quite easy to counter them.

See Appendix 4 for a complete list of arguments and how to counter them as well as advice from advocates on getting a school nutrition bill through the legislature.

Global Scene: UK Embarrassed into Action

Other countries face similar challenges when it comes to improving school food. But rapidly rising obesity rates among British children is now prompting serious action, in part thanks to celebrity chef Jamie Oliver's devastating 2005 television series on the sorry state of UK school meals. After Oliver gathered 270,000 signatures on his "Feed Me Better" petition and delivered them to Prime Minister Tony Blair, the government pledged an additional $500 million over three years to pay for such basics as kitchens and fresh ingredients for school meals. UK education secretary Ruth Kelly has also taken a strong stand on vending, pledging to ban foods high in fat, salt, and sugar by September 2006. Instead, vending machines will be expected to provide fresh fruit, milk, bottled water, and fruit juice. She declared that "the scandal of junk food served every day in school canteens must end."[33] Oliver is apparently setting his sights next on overhauling school food in the United States. We could use him.

Can We Get Out of This Mess?

No matter how hard the soda and junk food companies try to position themselves as being part of the solution, the truth is they care more about the health of their own bottom lines than that of children. Nowhere is this reality more evident than with school nutrition policy. Especially disturbing is how corporations such as Coca-Cola and PepsiCo are promoting their educational programs in the classroom (as described in Chapter 2) while also fighting to keep peddling their unhealthy products in the hallways.

Much is at stake in the battle over school food. It's clear that a grassroots movement is taking hold around the nation to improve school food. The good news is that this effort will continue unabated. It's even possible that industry will see the handwriting on the wall and eventually scale back its opposition in state legislatures. But how long will this take, and how many more resources will advocates require in the meantime? Even in California, it took six years to get compromised legislation passed. And many other states are just beginning their fights. Meanwhile, children continue to consume soda, chips, and cookies for lunch while the health effects mount. Can we really afford to wait for the slow, incremental legislative process to effect change? Secretly, some advocates tell me they are getting worn out. And who can blame them? How many times can you keep going up against Goliath before he wears you down?

Additional unanswered questions remain. Most of the advocacy efforts are focused on replacing junk food and sodas with supposedly healthier processed food and beverages. Because schools still rely on the money from competitive food sales, this strategy is being implemented as a compromise measure. But is it even possible to sell truly healthy food and beverages via vending machines? For example, in California, some schools are switching over to slightly improved, but still overly processed foods, such as granola bars and baked chips. Does this send children the best possible message about good nutrition? Also, what about the ethics of selling bottled water to children in poor inner-city schools? Why can't we invest in fixing water fountains so that all children can have free access to an essential human need?

The trouble with any solution short of doing away with school vending machines altogether is that we will remain mired in endless debate over what constitutes good nutrition. At the same time, as long we allow the same food and beverage companies to remain in schools, they will just develop new "approved" products to brand kids with. Or new rules will be ignored altogether. Or the entire movement will be co-opted as we saw with the voluntary agreement entered into by the soda industry with the Clinton Foundation in May 2006 (discussed in Chapter 1). Once the door is open, it becomes very tricky to enforce nutrition rules school by school, even where strong state laws get passed.

Moreover, focusing only on nutrition ignores all the other

ways in which corporations market to children in schools. Some groups concerned with more than just childhood obesity, such as the Campaign for a Commercial-Free Childhood and Commercial Alert, are calling for the complete removal of vending machines and all forms of marketing to children in schools. Why can't schools be the one safe haven left for children against the onslaught of corporate marketing?

Many nutrition advocates tell me that they would ideally like to get rid of vending machines altogether. However, they say, this position is just not politically tenable. Perhaps incremental change is the most viable strategy. But what if we shifted the conversation entirely? Instead of asking how schools can still make money by selling children slightly healthier food and beverages provided by corporations, how about we figure out how to serve healthy school meals and provide locally grown fresh fruit as snacks?

Many advocates are also working hard to improve school meals, for example, through innovative "farm-to-school" programs. We need to tie these efforts into larger conversations about corporate marketing in schools. Instead of asking what products Coca-Cola can sell that would pass nutrition muster, we should ask how we can properly fund public education so that we don't need Coca-Cola. Until we begin to truly value children and public education by asking these broader questions, the battles over school food will rage on.

Regulating Junk Food Marketing to Children

You want that nag factor so that seven-year-old Sarah is nagging Mom in the grocery stores to buy Funky Purple. We're not sure Mom would reach out for it on her own.[1]

—Kelly Stitt, senior brands manager, Heinz catsup division

Susan Linn is about the most mild-mannered, calm, and reasonable person you could ever meet. Not to mention, she has devoted her entire career to helping children. So it came as some surprise when the psychologist was called names like "clown," "idiot," "loser," and "fascist," and was told to "shut the hell up" in an onslaught of hate mail directed at her organization. Her crime? Daring to take on two popular corporations that target children with junk food advertising. That's how emotionally charged the issue has become in our national discourse.

When I think about how food companies target children, I

like to break it down into two categories: schools and every-where else. Nutrition advocates are trying to rid school vending machines of soda and junk food, but companies are lobbying hard against those efforts. The battle for "every-where else" creates its own set of challenges. Unlike schools, where tremendous grassroots momentum is building, the effort to address other forms of junk food marketing to chil-dren has been less successful—but not for lack of trying.

As concrete, four-walled institutions, schools are relatively straightforward targets for local or state policymaking. Also, legislation aimed at curbing exposure to junk food mar-keting in schools is unlikely to be controversial among par-ents or the public at large since most people agree that schools should be safe havens for children. Parents send their kids off to school with the expectation that other adults are acting on their behalf. In contrast, marketing that takes place outside of school is more associated with parental con-trol, making the idea of regulation more contentious. Another basic problem is that saturation advertising—conveyed through television, the Internet, video games, and other media—can be completely overwhelming. Where do we even begin? Such national forms of media for the most part require policymaking at the federal (and not simply the local or state) level.

Adding insult to injury, the federal government's conspic-uous reluctance to solve the problem has left advocates with few options other than to just keep complaining or initiate private litigation to try to fix it themselves. But that doesn't mean all is lost. Despite repeated attempts by government officials and food company executives to make excuses, such

as hiding behind the First Amendment's free speech protections, plenty of regulatory options exist.

As I started to learn more about this topic, I was struck by
the numerous misconceptions and myths being perpetuated.
It is vitally important to understand how the issues are being
framed, in order to further the dialogue and help lay the foundation for policy action. This chapter gets behind the anti-
regulatory rhetoric and points to other (hopefully more
useful) ways of talking about the important issue of junk food
marketing to children.

Problem? What Problem?

One of the food industry's favorite strategies is to deny that a
problem even exists. But when it comes to junk food marketing to children, the evidence is ubiquitous and unavoidable. The Center for Science in the Public Interest's excellent
2003 report, "Pestering Parents: How Food Companies
Market Obesity to Children," exposes the numerous strategies
industry uses to target kids.[2] Also, many advocacy groups,
such as the Campaign for a Commercial-Free Childhood and
Commercial Alert, have demanded congressional action, as
have prominent health organizations such as the American
Academy of Pediatrics, the American Public Health Association, and the American Psychological Association (APA).

The recommendations of APA's Task Force on Advertising
and Children are particularly compelling:

Considerable research has examined advertising's cumu-
lative effect on children's eating habits. Studies have documented that a high percentage of advertisements

targeting children feature candy, fast foods, and snacks and that exposure to such advertising increases consumption of these products. . . . Several studies have found strong associations between increases in advertising for nonnutritious foods and rates of childhood obesity. . . . We believe the accumulation of evidence on this topic is now compelling enough to warrant regulatory action by the government to protect the interests of children, and therefore offer a recommendation that restrictions be placed on advertising to children too young to recognize advertising's persuasive intent.[3]

Each year children see forty thousand television commercials, most of which are for unhealthy foods. But that's only the tip of the iceberg. Susan Linn author of *Consuming Kids*, starkly describes how technological advances—such as the Internet and cell phones—are exploited to bypass parents and target children directly.[4] Product placement (Coca-Cola merchandise on *American Idol*), cross promotions and movie tie-ins (*Star Wars* toy promotions at Burger King), brand licensing (Pop-Tarts boxes adorned with cartoon hero SpongeBob SquarePants), and marketing in schools all make television commercials seem tame by comparison.

Children are now marketed to in ways that were not contemplated even a few years ago. For example, "advergaming"— product promotion in video games—has become a permanent part of the marketing lexicon. Every major food company now uses this device, which is attractive to marketers given that the average amount of time a kid spends on a gaming Web site (twenty-six minutes) far exceeds the duration of a standard television commercial. Alarmed by this trend, advocacy groups negotiated a compromise in late 2005 with broadcasters and the Federal Communications Commission (FCC). The agreement is aimed at protecting children from "interactive television"—an emerging technology that promises, among other things, to give children the ability to order a pizza while watching TV. As Susan Linn notes: "TV commercials are so twentieth century. Marketers want to insinuate their brands into the hearts and minds of children."[5]

Moreover, young children have not developed the cognitive ability to even realize they are being marketed to. The exact cutoff age is the subject of some debate, but it's generally agreed that children under age eight cannot understand what experts call persuasive intent. And although older children usually understand what advertising is, they often lack the cognitive capacity to resist it.

The Verdict Is In: Guilty as Charged

Any lingering questions regarding the scientific connection between junk food marketing and children's health were put firmly to rest in late 2005 when a long-awaited report was released by the respected government advisory committee, the Institute of Medicine (IOM). The impressive five-hundred-page document—the collective effort of sixteen top-notch experts (including several from industry)—assessed the influence of food advertising directed at kids. Reviewing hundreds of studies, it found, rather unsurprisingly, that such marketing promotes preferences for high-calorie, low-nutrient foods and beverages, and encourages children to request and consume these products. While the committee said that no direct causal link has been established, it never-theless concluded that "the statistical association between ad viewing and obesity is strong" and that "even a small influ-ence would amount to a substantial impact when spread across the entire population."[6] Indeed, as Ellen Wartella, a member of the IOM committee (and advisor to Kraft Foods to boot) acknowledged: "We can't anymore argue whether food advertising is related to children's diets. It is."[7]

Government Has It Covered

It's no secret that the federal government has essentially thrown up its hands and abdicated all responsibility when it comes to reining in the out-of-control marketing of junk food to kids. Currently, federal laws to regulate marketing to children range from scant to nil. The FCC has jurisdiction over broadcasting and the Federal Trade Commission (FTC) is responsible for monitoring advertising. In the 1970s the FCC banned "host selling"—the embedding of commercials in children's program-ming. While this rule is still in effect today, it's hardly a formi-dable threat to advertisers, who can easily target young viewers of TV programs intended for adults. The most commonly cited example is Coca-Cola's product placement on *American Idol*, watched by millions of young children. Moreover, as Susan Linn notes, "given the increase in cross promotions and product licensing, de facto host selling is a component of almost all chil-dren's television."[8] In other words, kids' TV shows are effec-tively reduced to long commercials featuring beloved characters from the entertainment world. In lieu of adequate government regulation, industry has created a convenient solution doomed to failure: policing itself.

Self-regulation to the Rescue

When the issue of marketing to children started to really heat up in the 1970s, industry decided it better get proactive to avoid government meddling. So marketers created the self-regulatory body the Children's Advertising Review Unit (CARU). A program of the Council of Better Business Bureaus, CARU is charged with monitoring all national ads aimed at children age twelve and under.

Food-industry representatives love to point to CARU as doing a great job. While they might (under pressure) admit the agency could use a little tweak here and there, basically, the message is: we've got it covered, so government hands off.

Just one minor detail: the problem of junk food marketing to children has only gotten worse in the thirty years since CARU was established as the alternative to government action. Most experts agree with Senator Tom Harkin (one of the few children's champions left in Congress) when he says that self-regulation has been a complete failure:

> CARU, frankly, has become a poster child for how not to conduct self-regulation. Time and again, it has shown itself to be a captive of the industry. It has no real independence. No sanction authority. No teeth. The current situation is like a game with a rule book, but no real referee. CARU is a tiny group tasked with oversight of a multibillion-dollar industry. To me, the deck seems a bit stacked. And the proof is in the pudding. Look at the deluge of junk food advertising aimed at

kids that we see today. CARU has given the green light to all of it!⁹

Food law expert Ellen Fried, a researcher with the Rudd Center for Food Policy and Obesity at Yale University, agrees that CARU is largely ineffective, even when the agency tries to reprimand advertisers. "I've read enough case reports to see the same waltz repeatedly danced between CARU and food companies. All too often, CARU's admonishments have little effect on either the company's behavior or the harmful effects of advertising to children," she said. "As with all self-regulatory bodies, CARU is hampered by its being a creature of, and supported by, industry."¹⁰

Been There, Done That: A Brief History of Time

Too often issues are discussed without proper historical context. It's important to understand where we've been so we can have a clearer vision of where we are going. I have sat in enough meetings listening to current FTC officials saying that when it comes to regulating marketing to children, "we're not going there; we tried it before and it failed." I got so tired of hearing this sorry excuse that I decided to find out for myself what really happened. So let's set the historical record straight.

In 1978, the FTC attempted to pull in the reins on junk food marketing to kids with its infamous "Kid-Vid" initiative—which by today's standards was quite a radical undertaking. Tracy Westen was deputy director of the FTC's Bureau of Consumer Protection (under Chairman Michael Pertschuk's bold leadership) and in charge of the ill-fated proposal. At the time, the main health concern was dental cavities and the long-term impact of diets high in sugar. Chief among several agency objectives was advertising aimed at very young children, up to age six, who couldn't even understand what ads were. The FTC proposal included banning all TV ads to young children and banning ads for highly sugared products aimed at older kids, the theory being that even older kids lack the ability to understand serious long-term health consequences. Other ideas were to limit specific messages and reduce the total number of ads.

Westen strongly believed (and still does) that advertising to very young children is wrong. He says that while the agency concluded that young kids were deceived by TV advertising, the difficulty was in drafting a workable remedy, because kids and adults watch TV together.

Three years later, the FTC terminated the effort without taking any action. What happened in between was an unfortunate combination of politics and bad timing. The advertising industry raised $16 million to lobby against the rulemaking, an amount equal to one-quarter of the FTC's budget at the time.[11]

During a tumultuous three-year period, the FTC was put through the political wringer, an ordeal that included a federal court's decision to disqualify FTC chairman Michael Pertschuk for being biased. Although he was later reinstated on First Amendment grounds, the chairman ultimately recused himself from the proceedings under political pressure. The FTC also endured:

- Being called a "national nanny" in a *Washington Post* editorial
- Congress stripping the commission of part of its

jurisdiction over marketing aimed at children—a loss of authority that persists to this day

- The passage of a congressional bill allowing the House and Senate to veto any rule making by the agency (legislation that was later overturned by the Supreme Court)

- President Ronald Reagan's appointment of Republican James Miller as FTC chair (Miller was committed to ending the commission's rule-making authority)[12]

Westen says that the political fallout was a surprise to everyone: "Nobody saw it coming. The rulemaking was seen as attacking a broad range of industry groups. Even the tobacco industry was opposed because they figured they would be regulated next. Ultimately, the initiative's failure wasn't for First Amendment reasons, and it wasn't because we concluded that kids aren't deceived," he said. Rather, it was due to the overwhelming negative reaction from Congress and its high-powered corporate allies.

Westen explains that by the end of the 1970s, the heyday of Ralph Nader was passing and a new political climate was emerging: "It was clear to the staff that politically the proposed rule was not going forward. If Congress and the commission had been pushing us to pass it, we might have come to a different conclusion."[13]

So, Westen left Washington and returned to California to start a nonprofit, the Center for Governmental Studies, which focuses on campaign-finance reform. "I still think we were right in principle," he says, "but way ahead of our time. The arguments for some regulation of children's TV advertising were very compelling. People assumed the remedies would never work, but the fact that other countries have done it shows that it's doable." Westen thinks that the reason the FTC has been loath to take action ever since is that the agency is gun-shy. "I think people felt burned by the political fallout and aren't willing to touch it again."

So the next time you hear a federal government official try to claim that the 1970s effort to regulate junk food marketing to kids "didn't work," don't believe it. With a strong enough political will to overcome corporate forces, it certainly could.

Debunking the Myth of the First Amendment

The most common myth perpetuated by ad agencies and their food-industry clients is that free speech guaranteed by the First Amendment is an impenetrable legal barrier to the federal government's ability to curtail advertising aimed at children. Indeed, advertisers used the First Amendment as a shield against the irrefutable and damning research findings by the Institute of Medicine described earlier. Feeling threatened by the IOM's quite tame recommendation that Congress take action if food companies didn't shape up within two years, Dan Jaffe, the executive vice president for government relations (aka lobbying) at the Association of National Advertisers said:

> We were deeply disappointed by the IOM's call for congressional action to mandate a specific shift in the way companies allocate their ad spending. This is a radical and unconstitutional proposal that would have

an impact far beyond food advertising. It not only is contrary to good policy, but most certainly would violate the First Amendment.[14]

That's pretty strong language, but it amounts to a lot of hot air. (Not to mention, a constitutional law scholar from Yale Law School was a member of the IOM committee.) To make matters worse, federal government officials disinclined to rattle corporate cages also perpetuate the legend of free speech protection.

For example, current FTC chairperson Deborah Platt Majoras set the stage quite starkly in her opening remarks to a 2005 FTC meeting on food marketing to children: "We are well aware that some are already calling on government to regulate rather than facilitate. From the FTC's perspective, we believe a ban on children's advertising is neither wise nor viable."[15] By "not viable," Majoras meant that such regulation wouldn't pass First Amendment muster.

This myth has been so widely disseminated that I have even heard colleagues repeat it as truth. But legal concepts are rarely black-and-white. (Why else would we need so many lawyers?) A closer look at First Amendment law reveals many more shades of gray. All rights must be balanced against competing societal interests. And that's where constitutional interpretation can get quite murky.

Corporate advertising falls under what's called "commercial speech," a category that actually enjoys less constitutional protection than the broader category of "free speech," the kind normally associated with individuals and the press. Government restrictions on commercial advertising can indeed be constitutional, as long as they meet the legal test established by the Supreme Court.

It's true that in recent years the Supreme Court has gravitated toward a more strict interpretation of the commercial speech doctrine, and has thus been loath to allow too much government restriction of advertising. Most notably, in 2001, the Court declared unconstitutional a Massachusetts law banning, among other things, outdoor tobacco advertising within 1,000 feet of schools or playgrounds. (The state's intent was to protect children from tobacco ads.) The Court said the law was too broad because it would restrict not only children's but adults' access to information. (Of course, whether adults really need "access" to tobacco advertising is another story.) This decision—known as *Lorillard v. Reilly*—has since been exaggerated by food companies eager to claim a sacrosanct First Amendment right to advertise anything, anywhere, anytime.

But we shouldn't be intimidated by industry arguments that this case establishes a legal precedent against regulations on junk food marketing to children. In fact, the decision tells us very little about how the Court might rule, because the Massachusetts law it overturned barred advertising directed at *adults*. In other words, laws designed to curb ads that target kids exclusively (those appearing on children's television, for instance) have not yet been tested against the Court's commercial speech analysis.

Moreover, plenty of legal experts don't buy the line that the First Amendment is a barrier to regulation, especially in protecting young children. Former FTC staffer Tracy Westen says that ads aimed at young children are inherently deceptive and as such are not entitled to free speech protection under the First Amendment.[16]

Angela Campbell, a professor at Georgetown University Law Center and an expert in children's media, agrees. Campbell has proposed a federal ban on the use of cartoon characters to hawk junk food, along with product placement in movies and TV programs aimed at children. Like Westen, she maintains that such techniques are intrinsically manipulative and therefore do not deserve First Amendment free speech protection.[17]

So don't let food companies, marketers, and government officials wrap themselves in the Constitution. All the rhetoric really amounts to is a convenient excuse that covers up a self-serving desire to maintain the status quo.

Is this what the founding fathers really meant by free speech?

While it's true that the current Supreme Court has shown a willingness to grant corporations limited free speech protection, you might be wondering, how can this be? How did corporations gain access to a set of rights that were originally intended for individuals? Good question. Unfortunately, I can offer no easy answer. Indeed, many experts question the very idea of so-called legal personhood, a nineteenth-century doctrine that grants corporations constitutional protections otherwise enjoyed only by actual people.

Whose interests exactly are we defending when we allow corporations to benefit from "free speech" protection? To quote *Food Politics* author Marion Nestle, "I'm having a hard time believing that the founding fathers had in mind advertising to children when they wrote the First Amendment to the

Constitution."[18] It is difficult indeed to imagine that the same free speech guarantees that allowed the *New York Times* to publish the Pentagon Papers should also be extended to advertisements for Cap'n Crunch and Count Chocula cereals.

Why We Can't Sugarcoat a Sugary Mess

One of the more frustrating aspects of talking about food marketing aimed at kids is how the dialogue has been completely twisted to benefit industry. What started out as complaints being leveled at companies for how they are marketing the wrong kinds of foods has turned into talking about how they can market the "right" kinds.

Indeed, this was the focus at the July 2005 FTC workshop on "self-regulation" and food marketing mentioned previously. One by one, industry executives proclaimed what a great job they were doing at marketing allegedly healthier foods to kids. Even academic experts opined maddeningly about how we should encourage industry to put its immense marketing ingenuity and resources to good use.

But this narrow framing and wishful thinking conveniently ignores the 800-pound gorilla in the room. How can we begin to discuss eating the right food unless and until we talk about controlling an industry that spends billions of dollars a year trying to get children to eat the wrong food?

Also disappointing was a recommendation in the 2005 IOM report mentioned earlier that food companies "develop and promote healthier products." The IOM also stressed the need for more government funding of "social marketing," campaigns designed to promote healthy eating, such as the National Cancer Institute's "5 a Day" program.[19]

While it's true that government programs to promote fruits and vegetables pale in comparison to the marketing budgets of most corporations,[20] a little more funding from Uncle Sam is hardly going to make a dent. As former HHS secretary Tommy Thompson himself noted, "It's impossible to be in balance—the government is not going to spend that kind of money."[21] Moreover, recent corporate efforts to emblazon packages of spinach and carrots with much-loved cartoon figures like SpongeBob SquarePants can't hold a candle to the full-throttle deployment of those same characters in the service of junk food marketing.

What's Left? Sue the Bastards

When all other policy avenues—i.e., government regulation, legislation, and industry self-regulation—have been exhausted, one legal option remains: litigation. Groups such as CSPI, which has grown increasingly frustrated with inaction on the part of federal regulators, are turning to the court system for relief. As CSPI's litigation director Steve Gardner says, "Lawsuits are not the best way to resolve a dispute, but sometimes they are the only way."[22]

In January 2006, CSPI and the Campaign for a Commercial-Free Childhood (CCFC) announced their intention to sue Kellogg and Viacom (the parent company of Nickelodeon) for marketing junk food to children. The aim is to enjoin these companies from marketing junk foods where 15 percent or more of the target audience is composed of children under age eight.

While it's understandable that consumer groups would turn to the courts as a last resort, the idea of suing the creators of such family favorites as Tony the Tiger and SpongeBob SquarePants can be a tough sell to the general public. Indeed, upon announcing the lawsuit, both groups were vehemently attacked in the media and by the public for filing such a "frivolous" claim. My colleagues at CCFC shared some of the many angry e-mail messages they received (a few name-calling examples were listed at the start of this chapter). I was frankly astonished at the level of misunderstanding of the case. The most common complaint was that parents were "abdicating" their responsibility. But as CSPI's Gardner responded: "Parents are also responsible for making sure their young kids don't get hit by cars. But if someone's recklessly driving around your neighborhood at eighty miles an hour, you're going to want to stop them."[23]

In other words, parents are doing the best they can in a world that makes it almost impossible to protect their children. Our society has created a set of laws designed to protect consumers from harm. And filing a lawsuit is one of the few ways that private citizens have of enforcing those laws. So, if the law says that marketing to a young child is deceptive because she is too young to understand, why shouldn't we apply that law, even to Tony the Tiger?

Helping Parents Fight Back

Blaming parents is one of the food industry's favorite ways of absolving itself of responsibility for the problems it has caused. At the 2005 FTC workshop on advertising and childhood obesity, the federal government showed its true colors by dutifully playing industry's blame game, calling on parents to be more "responsible" in resisting junk food marketing. For example, Surgeon General Richard Carmona said, "We must remember that the best role models children have are their parents."[24] Panelist Margo Wootan, director of nutrition policy for the CSPI, has heard this line before. She boldly stood up for parents at the meeting with this response:

> If you listen to industry and government officials talk about parental responsibility, parents are supposed to work with their school boards to get soda and junk food out of schools, we're supposed to get fast-food companies to provide nutrition information, we're supposed to work with multibillion-dollar, multinational corporations to get them to change their marketing practices, all while we take care our family, take care of our home, and work full-time. Let's talk about parental responsibility, but let's put it in the context of what parents are facing, the resources and the expertise they have. This is crazy, what we are asking them to do. Today's parents are completely outmaneuvered by food marketers. Getting our children to eat a healthy diet would be much easier if we didn't have to contend with billions of dollars' worth of marketing for mostly nutritionally deficient foods.[25]

Amen. Here are some other ways to counter the parental responsibility argument.[26]

Yes, parents have a role to play, but so do corporations
Of course parents have an important and critical role to play

in teaching their children good eating habits and in modeling that behavior. However, food corporations spend roughly $12 billion a year directly targeting children with junk food marketing. What responsibility do corporations have to not undermine parental responsibility? As Senator Tom Harkin has aptly noted:

> No question, many parents need to make better choices for their children. They need to say no. But there are practical limits on what we can expect. It is just not realistic to think that most parents are going to deny their children access to TV on Saturday morning and after school. And, for goodness sake, why do we have a situation where conscientious parents have to protect their children from the ads on Saturday-morning TV?[27]

Companies bypass parents and market directly to kids

Advertisements are often designed to encourage children to beg their parents by buy junk food (known in the trade as the "nag factor"). Nagging and other marketing-driven behaviors threaten to undermine parental authority. Talk to any parent who has tried to survive a trip to the grocery store with young children in tow and you will understand how difficult it is to compete with omnipresent messages from food marketers. A stroll down the cereal aisle, for example, inevitably brings kids face to face with products deliberately and enticingly positioned at their eye level. It's disingenuous for companies to talk about parental responsibility while they deliberately target kids.

Corporations use highly specialized marketing tactics

Several times a year, a trade conference aptly named "Kid Power" showcases the latest techniques for marketing to children. At the February 2006 meeting, junk food peddlers learned countless tricks of the trade at workshops such as "Character Development to Create an Emotional Connection" and "Utilizing Branding to Create Increased Value Perception among Kids in School Cafeterias." How is a parent supposed to compete with all of that psychological marketing savvy?

Messages that reinforce the druglike effects of eating junk food are another favorite marketing technique. In her book *Born to Buy*, Juliet Schor explains how Cheetos advertisements cheerfully acknowledge the connection, "warning" that consumption of the neon-orange nuggets could result in "signs of cheese-crazed behavior" and leave the eater "officially hooked." The only cure: "a never-ending supply of that cheesy crunch you crave." Advertisers have made similar claims for products high in caffeine and/or sugar. Schor concludes that "companies are skirting dangerously close to a subtle association with drugs."[28]

It's not just food that's the problem

Of course it's not only junk food marketing that parents must contend with, but also advertising for toys, video games, clothing, CDs, cell phones, computers—you name it. So parents are placed in the unenviable position of having to regularly do battle with their own children. Why have we accepted at face value a society in which the concerns of parents are continuously pitted against the market-generated consumption demands of their kids?

An epidemic of bad parenting?

Has something drastic happened to parenting skills in recent years? Has a sudden outbreak of parental irresponsibility taken hold of the nation, precipitating a rise in childhood obesity and other problems over which parents were once firmly in control? In the vivid imagination of food marketers, the rise in childhood obesity can only be explained by bad parenting.

Protecting children in other ways

Most people recognize that powerful business forces sometimes need to be constrained by government intervention. We don't view laws banning alcohol, tobacco, and pornography sales to minors, for example, as usurpations of parental authority or a sign of a governmental nanny state. If anything, such restrictions encourage parents to be even more vigilant about their kids' use of these products. In other words, these laws help parents to be good parents.

Global Solutions Outdo Uncle Sam

The U.S. federal government's hands-off policy toward corporate marketers is especially disappointing when you consider how other countries are tackling the problem. A 2004 survey by the World Health Organization found that 85 percent of seventy-three countries impose some form of regulation on television advertising to children.[29]

In 1980, for example, Quebec became the first jurisdiction in the world to ban nearly all commercial advertising aimed at children. For more than twenty-five years, the Canadian province has had a comprehensive legislative ban on advertising to children under age thirteen. The law was motivated partly by public health concerns, but its principal aim is to protect a uniquely vulnerable group—children— from marketing manipulation. To get around the prohibition, advertisers in Quebec have targeted parents instead with ads for child-oriented products.[30] Imagine, the sky didn't fall; instead, marketers simply adjusted their practices accordingly.

Also, Sweden banned all television and radio advertising aimed at kids under age twelve in 1991. The law was enacted due to the concern that younger children couldn't clearly distinguish advertising from other programming. Also, policy makers believed that children should have the right to grow up in a commercial-free environment.[31] Now that's common-sense reasoning that we could use over here. Norway enacted a similar ban in 1992.

In Ireland, all television commercials for fast food and candy are banned. However, children are not spared from commercials emanating from satellite television channels from the United States and the United Kingdom. Broadcasts from other countries without similar restrictions are presenting ongoing dilemmas to nations trying to protect their children. Such increasing "cross-border" challenges suggest that we need to tackle this issue at the global level.

Critics of restrictions on junk food marketing to kids are quick to deny that initiatives like these are having any impact on childhood obesity. For example, the libertarian Cato Institute insists that:

Ad bans have failed everywhere they've been tried. So far, the list includes Sweden, Quebec, and Norway. None of these places have shown comparatively significant reductions in child obesity. In Sweden, the restrictions have been in place for a decade, yet the country's childhood obesity rates are in line with the rest of Europe's.[32]

This disingenuous argument is handily countered by Neville Rigby, director of policy and public affairs for the International Obesity Taskforce. Rigby says that it's "quite willfully misleading" for industry to claim that restrictions in other countries don't work. He says that rates of childhood obesity are indeed lower in countries with restrictions. By comparison, "UK children are exposed to more food advertising than others in Europe and have rapidly increasing levels of overweight and obesity." And this is true even though existing bans were not designed to protect children from obesity per se but to shield them from predatory marketers. In any case, says Rigby, industry efforts to disavow the possibility of an association between advertising regulations and lower rates of obesity are deceptive: "The fact is, no country has a complete ban on food marketing to children and there are no designed studies to measure the effects in this way."[33]

Corinna Hawkes, author of the landmark World Health Organization study that reviewed seventy-five countries' regulations on food marketing, agrees with Rigby. "It is very difficult to measure the effects of a ban on obesity because of all the other confounding factors," she says. "But that does not mean we can't make intelligent judgments based on the evidence available on advertising and food choices." The problem, she says, is that the lack of perfect evidence is exploited by the food industry. "They say that obesity in Sweden proves that banning advertising will fail to prevent obesity, when in fact there is no proof either way." Hawkes acknowledges that a ban is not the "magic bullet." "But who is claiming it is?" she says. "Industry is twisting the arguments in a completely hypocritical way."[34]

According to Richard Daynard, the cigarette industry also tried to claim for years that marketing restrictions had no impact. That ruse was put to rest when in 1999 the World Bank conducted a definitive study showing that tobacco ad bans really did reduce smoking. The research concluded that "bans on advertising and promotion prove effective, but only if they are comprehensive, covering all media and all uses of brand names and logos."[35] Indeed, the evidence suggests the need to impose more, not fewer, restrictions on reckless corporate marketing to protect public health.

Can Anything Be Done?

People (especially parents) invariably ask me: what can we do? I must admit this is a tough question for me to answer. While there are ways that parents can try to limit their children's exposure to marketing, obviously you can't lock your kids up in their rooms or blindfold them when they visit their friends' houses. So mostly, just do the best you can by talking to them about how marketing is deceptive and manipulative. Most kids don't like to be lied to and can understand this concept. Ultimately, though, we need to work toward policy-based solutions.

In thinking about the numerous ways that kids are bombarded with marketing messages, it can seem overwhelming to know where to even begin. Let's start with how the federal government could regulate. One way is to restore the FTC's full authority over food advertising aimed at children, as Senator Tom Harkin proposes in his Healthy Lifestyles and Prevention (HeLP) America Act.[36]

This far-ranging legislation would also give the secretary of agriculture the ability to prohibit the marketing and advertising of junk food in schools participating in school lunch or breakfast programs. The bill would also require the USDA to update its definition of foods of minimal nutritional value, which has not changed in more than thirty years, to conform to current nutrition science. And, if enacted, the law would require nutritional information on menus of chain restaurants.

All of these ideas are excellent and would certainly help rein in junk food marketing to children. It's especially appealing to address these issues at the national level because of the inefficiency of trying to pass bills state by state, not to mention one school district at a time. However, for the time being at least, the politics may be insurmountable.

That's why another policy option some advocates are talking about is local and community-based solutions to limit children's exposure to junk food marketing. For example, you could have local zoning laws to restrict the location of fast-food outlets within a certain distance from a school. Such laws have been used to regulate the sale of tobacco products under the same child-protection theory. Another idea is to pass a local ordinance that would ban the use of toys to sell food. (I am a particular fan of this idea and would love to see it implemented.) One major advantage of these ideas is that they don't restrict advertising per se, so are less likely to run the risk of a First Amendment challenge from industry.[37]

Another major advantage is that ideas like zoning laws and toy bans can be more easily accomplished at the local level, which is where most tobacco control policies have had the most success. Ultimately, such a strategy can create a grassroots movement that bubbles up to the state and even federal levels. The best analogy is how in California, cities started passing clean indoor air laws to protect workers and patrons from secondhand smoke, eventually resulting in a statewide law that has served as a model for other states around the nation.

We're also likely to see litigation as an increasing strategy, given the limited options available to make change happen on a broader scale. Ultimately, however, such approaches, as innovative as they might be, are going to seem meager in comparison with the vast resources at industry's disposal.

Much of the debate around this issue will likely continue to revolve around the science and what policy makers still perceive as questions related to the connection between junk food marketing and childhood obesity. The damning 2005 Institute of Medicine report should have put an end to scientific debate once and for all. And yet, the silence among federal policy makers in the wake of the report's release is deafening. Where are the congressional hearings? Why are we even still talking about self-regulation as the answer? We need no further proof that it's politics and not science that's driving this debate.

To me, the question comes down to morality more than science. It's not just about the health manifestations associated with kids eating too much junk food. As other countries have recognized, children should not be exploited for commercial gain, no matter the reason. That's why we need a broader discussion related to protecting the most vulnerable members of our society. Don't children deserve to grow up in a world where they aren't constantly targeted as little consumers?

12

Scapegoating Lawyers

This is a solution in search of a problem.[1]
—Wisconsin governor Jim Doyle vetoing legislation
to shield industry from obesity lawsuits

Growing up in a low-income section of New York City, Jazlyn Bradley, by the age of nineteen, had been eating McDonald's food for her entire life. As frequently as five times a week, her diet consisted of McMuffins for breakfast, Chicken McNuggets for lunch, and Big Macs for dinner. As a child, she loved collecting the Happy Meal toys. Compared to her run-down home, which lacked even a kitchen sink, McDonald's was a comfortable, clean, and safe place to eat.

Jazlyn Bradley and others like her are named in a class action lawsuit that blames the fast-food giant for misrepresenting its products as nutritious and for not revealing potential hazards. At the time of filing in 2002, Jazlyn weighed 270 pounds and was diagnosed with diabetes, hypertension, and high cholesterol—maladies usually associated with middle age. Bradley's father, Israel, a single parent, said he never saw anything in the restaurants that informed him of the food's ingredients. "I always believed McDonald's was healthy for my children," he said in an affidavit.[2]

While this widely misunderstood case remains the only one of its kind filed anywhere in the nation, the corporate backlash has resulted in a serious threat to consumers' ability to seek redress through the court system. In Congress and state legislatures around the country, bills are being proposed to shield the food industry from allegedly "frivolous" lawsuits related to obesity. With names like the "Commonsense Consumption Act," such bills have already passed in twenty-one states and are pending in about a dozen more at this writing.

A federal version of the law passed the House twice (2004 and 2005) by an overwhelming margin each time and is still pending in the Senate, where its chances are less certain. If enacted, the legislation would preemptively shield all sectors of the food industry from lawsuits brought for obesity or obesity-related health problems and would apply to cases brought in either federal or state court.

When industry is under attack, a critical part of their strategy for fighting back is to go on the offensive by pushing for legislation that protects their collective interests.

Earlier, I explained efforts by industry to *oppose* legislation intended to advance public health; these bills are a rare example of *proactive* nutrition-related legislation by industry. In this chapter, we will witness the food industry's hardball lobbying tactics being brought to an all-time low. Through a combination of trumped-up hysteria, scapegoating, and downright dishonesty, the food industry is seizing the opportunity to spin this nonissue to maximum PR advantage. As such, it's the ultimate hypocrisy: while food companies are busy proclaiming how much they want to be part of the solution, behind the scenes, they are lobbying to protect themselves from potential liability against health-related claims. Instead of cleaning up their act to avoid becoming a target of litigation, they're aiming to insulate themselves in perpetuity by strong-arming the legislative process. This chapter explains what's at stake, who is behind the effort, and how you can counter the corporate rhetoric.

STATES WITH LAWS THAT BAN OBESITY LAWSUITS

Arizona, Colorado, Florida, Georgia, Idaho, Illinois, Kansas, Kentucky, Louisiana, Maine, Michigan, Missouri, North Dakota, Ohio, Oregon, South Dakota, Utah, Tennessee, Texas, Washington, and Wyoming.

(as of March 2006)

A Solution in Search of a Problem

The media loves to cover "David vs. Goliath" lawsuits, especially when the target is a well-known company such as McDonald's. As food companies come under increasing attack for their unhealthy products and overzealous marketing, the media seizes on every opportunity to talk about the idea of suing Big Food. Of course, an important industry goal is to avoid becoming a target for litigation. While the lobbying effort to shield food companies from legal liability fits squarely into this aim, here's a dirty little secret that corporate lobbyists and their puppet politicians don't want you to know: there is no need for these bills. Industry has created a solution to a problem that doesn't exist.

Capitalizing on excessive media coverage, lobbyists give the false impression that poor restaurants are practically on the verge of bankruptcy thanks to the nefarious efforts of an army of greedy trial lawyers, and that legislators must act quickly to stop the bleeding. But while there has been much talk of litigation as a way to hold some food companies accountable, it's still mostly just talk. In addition, current safeguards already protect against baseless lawsuits.

And yet the lobbying effort has mushroomed into a state-by-state onslaught that borders on the absurd. For example, South Dakota is even protecting local ranchers of obscure animals such as bison and ostriches. Not to be outdone, New Mexico's bill is called the "Right to Eat Enchiladas Act" and Wyoming is curiously protecting homeless shelters, soup kitchens, and food banks.

The long-term strategy is to protect Big Food from the fate of the major tobacco companies who ultimately became vulnerable in the courtroom. "We need to take steps to make sure that the restaurant industry doesn't become the next Big Tobacco,"[3] explained Bryan Malenius, chief of staff for Representative Ric Keller (R-FL). Keller is the author of the federal bill and acknowledged fast-food fan whose top donors include Outback Steakhouse and the National Beer Wholesalers Association. But in the short term, this issue is really just a smokescreen.

Despite all the finger-pointing at greedy trial lawyers, the first case against McDonald's that actually made a health-related claim was thrown out by the trial court. The same lawyer then filed a class action on behalf of children (the Jazlyn Bradley case), which was at first dismissed by the trial court. In January 2005, an appeals court overturned part of that decision, sending it back to the trial level. This is where things stand as of spring 2006. So, we still don't even know yet whether this case will ultimately be successful. Yet industry acts like the sky is falling.

Wisconsin governor Jim Doyle said it best as he vetoed the bill in his state to outlaw such suits: "This is a solution in search of a problem, and is not needed. I have great confidence that our judges and juries will respect the law and apply common sense and quickly dismiss any frivolous litigation."[4]

Why You Should Care, Even If You Hate Lawyers

Maybe you're wondering: who doesn't know by now, especially with the success of the documentary *Super Size Me*, that eating too much fast food isn't good for you? Why should food companies be held responsible by people who lack common sense or don't have enough willpower? Is litigation really the answer to solving America's obesity epidemic? I have asked myself all of these questions.

Even as a lawyer, litigation is not my preferred strategy for social change, mainly because it comes too late—compensating victims long after the damage is already done, doing little to prevent harm from occurring in the first place.

However, I still believe that the right to sue should be preserved, for several reasons. For one, litigation can often play an important role in public policy. As we have seen throughout this book, industry is very effective at lobbying to prevent legislation to improve nutrition and public health. Litigation can scare industry into improving its behavior, while bypassing politicized legislative channels. Litigation can also bring an important issue into the public eye, which in turn puts pressure on legislators. A good example is how, in the tobacco wars, lawsuits helped shift public sentiment and this led to legislative action.

The courtroom is the last resort

Also, the courtroom is often a consumer's last resort for holding corporations accountable. In today's political climate, all other legal avenues are failing to protect public health: the federal government is feeble, state legislation is being undermined by corporate lobbying, and industry self-regulation is a joke. This leaves only one remaining option: litigation. Here's another way to look at it. Under the U.S. system, we have three branches of government: executive (the president and regulatory agencies), legislative (Congress and states), and judicial (the court system). With the first two branches having failed us, all we have left is the third. If this option gets shut down, there is nowhere else to turn.

Food companies don't deserve special treatment

Another reason we should protect the individual's right to sue is simple justice. It's unfair for one particular industry to carve out an exception for itself. Why should consumers be able to sue automobile manufacturers, chemical companies, the pharmaceutical industry, etc., but not Big Food? There is nothing inherent about food that makes it any less subject to a system of laws that are designed to protect consumers from wrongdoing by any industry. These laws have evolved over the past century and are firmly entrenched in our legal system. In legalese, it's called civil justice. It's the height of arrogance for food-industry lobbyists to attempt to override the current civil justice system by passing new laws that would make corporations unaccountable.

Also, over the past several decades, food processing has become highly industrialized, resulting in increased hazards in the food supply, including biological pathogens and cancer-causing chemicals. The days of cooking up a batch of soup in your mother's kitchen are fast disappearing, being replaced by assembly-line factory production. Why should manufacturers who have created this industrialized food-production system be exempted from consumer-protection laws designed to apply to all potential bad corporate actors?

Food companies hide information and mislead customers

In attempting to shield itself from liability, food-industry rhetoric rests on the questionable assumption that anyone who consumes its products is *fully informed* of the risks of doing so. This position further presupposes that food companies have actually *disclosed* all the pertinent information. However, as we've seen, the same industry that touts "consumer education" as a solution to obesity has also blocked every effort to require nutrition labeling in chain restaurants. This "failure to disclose" (in legal jargon) is a critical component of the New York lawsuit brought against McDonald's.

For example, lawyers argued that McDonald's failed to advise customers of risks that were not common knowledge and failed to warn that eating fattening foods can cause addictive effects similar to nicotine—two serious charges. In his initial decision, which indicated some sympathy with the plaintiff's case, the judge described Chicken McNuggets as follows: "Rather than being merely chicken fried in a pan, [they] are a McFrankenstein creation of various elements not utilized by the home cook."[5] Next the judge listed the rather lengthy and strange-sounding ingredients contained in a Chicken McNugget, which are, in addition to chicken:

Water, salt, modified corn starch, sodium phosphates, chicken broth powder (chicken broth, salt and natural flavoring [chicken source]), seasoning (vegetable oil, extracts of rosemary, mono, di- and triglycerides, lecithin). Battered and breaded with water, enriched bleached wheat flour (niacin, iron, thiamine, mononitrate, riboflavin, folic acid), yellow corn flour, bleached wheat flour, modified corn starch, salt, leavening (baking soda, sodium acid pyrophosphate, sodium aluminum phosphate, monocalcium phosphate, calcium lactate), spices, wheat starch, dried whey, corn starch. Batter set in vegetable shortening. Cooked in partially hydrogenated vegetable oils (may contain partially hydrogenated soybean oil and/or partially hydrogenated corn oil and/or partially hydrogenated canola oil and/or cottonseed oil and/or corn oil). TBHQ and citric acid added to help preserve freshness. Dimethylpolysiloxane added as an anti-foaming agent.[6]

Because consumers are often left in the dark, resulting in potential untoward consequences, the court system provides a way to shine a light on hidden corporate practices while compensating victims. And, if you're wondering how these ingredients could possibly be harmful, since they had to pass muster with the U.S. Food and Drug Administration, such government oversight has long been criticized as inadequate. This is precisely why we need litigation as a fall-back plan, for when other regulatory mechanisms fail to operate properly.

Also, believe it or not, there was a time when McDonald's marketed its food as healthful, long before salads were ever added to the menu. Claiming that cheeseburgers and fries are nutritious may seem laughable by today's standards, but it's true. The media spin about the McDonald's case is that it's simply about getting fat from eating too much fast food. Ellen Fried, who teaches food law at New York University, says the lawsuit is not about obesity per se, but rather about deceptive advertising and how McDonald's was advertising its food as nutritious. "You have to go back a couple of years, before all the attention to this issue got started. Most people didn't think that going to McDonald's daily was a problem. It was advertised as healthful, perfectly OK to eat every day and supersize it and eat more. You have to ask what responsibility McDonald's has to its customers. Obviously, they can't lie or present information in a deceptive way. It's not about 'I ate this and it made me fat,' it's about what you told me about eating this way, or didn't tell me."[7]

Liability protection in perpetuity

Finally and most dramatically, passage of these laws has

serious potential to shield industry from any future liability, thereby rendering food companies completely unaccountable to the public—forever. We have no idea what additional scientific evidence could be discovered down the road that might shed a whole new light on corporate accountability. There was a time when people thought it was crazy to sue tobacco companies. Then scientific research into the addictive nature of nicotine changed everything. If we allow industry to shield itself from liability now, we are closing the door to future potential legitimate claims, which is of course exactly what industry wants.

Mindy Kursban, executive director and general counsel for Physicians' Committee for Responsible Medicine (who is suing the Atkins estate, demanding labels warning of hazards of the heavily meat-centered diet) says these bills are dangerously premature. "Questions regarding the role of the food industry in our nation's obesity epidemic are just now being brought to light. Rather than immediately absolve the entire industry of all potential liability, we should learn more about how they have contributed to this public health crisis," she said.[8]

Of course, that's the last thing industry wants—to be held responsible. So corporate lobbyists have created an imaginary threat based on one unresolved lawsuit and are convincing sympathetic politicians to pass new laws to essentially undo an entire legal system of consumer protection.

It's the Documents, Stupid

Why is industry so determined to shield itself from liability if there's no real risk?

Whether or not it makes sense for someone who eats too

many Big Macs to sue McDonald's is really beside the point to industry. What scares food companies even more than costly jury verdicts is the prospect of the discovery process (when lawyers are allowed access to the defendant's documents and other inside information) unearthing damning information about dishonest industry practices. This, in turn, can open the door to a plethora of new government regulations.

An avalanche of damning documents discovered through litigation against the tobacco industry revealed so much information that an entire research group in California is dedicated to its study.[9] This irrefutable trail of industry malfeasance was critical to shifting public opinion against Big Tobacco. The food industry has learned from tobacco that litigation is a powerful public interest tool.

Just what exactly could be revealed through litigation that might harm Big Food? One possibility is evidence of efforts to addict consumers. According to information uncovered by the Physicians Committee for Responsible Medicine, some manufacturers deliberately target consumers who are vulnerable to certain food addictions. For example, research suggests that some of the least healthy foods—such as chocolate, sugar, meat, and cheese—are physically addictive.[10] Another study comparing PET scans of people on cocaine with people who overate resulted in similar brain patterns for the two groups. Overeaters also demonstrate typical addiction behaviors such as cravings and loss of control.[11]

Lawsuits could help uncover the extent to which the food industry knew about, concealed, and took advantage of food addictions. Given how the tobacco industry covered up its knowledge of nicotine's addictiveness for decades, the parallels are potentially ominous. That explains in part why the restaurant industry and food manufacturers have teamed up to keep potentially damning evidence from being used against them. To better understand why industry is so focused on passing these bills, I decided to go to the source.

In the Belly of the Beast

In September 2004, I attended a conference called "Legal and Strategic Guide to Minimizing Liability for Obesity: What Food Industry Counsel Need to Know Now." It was sponsored by the notorious tobacco defense law firm Jones Day. The roughly 100 attendees included lawyers and other representatives of all the top food companies, such as McDonald's, Kraft Foods, Mars, PepsiCo, Yum Brands (which owns Taco Bell, KFC, and Pizza Hut), Kellogg, Coca-Cola, and Altria, the tobacco company formerly known as Philip Morris.

If you're wondering how an outspoken nutrition advocate and industry critic got in, I simply asked for and received press credentials. (As a writer, I make such requests all the time.) But within the first few minutes of the meeting, it was clear that somebody had made a mistake. The attendees were assured that it was a "closed conference," with no one from the plaintiffs' side having been invited, and thus everyone could speak freely. I never misrepresented myself, but I felt like a spy, and enjoyed every minute of it.

In one presentation, called "Lessons Learned from Tobacco," Jones Day attorney Paul Crist explained how the advocates were comparing food companies to the tobacco industry. I almost jumped out of my skin when he displayed excerpts of an article that I wrote entitled "Big Food Lawsuits Can Help Trim America's Waistline." You know you're having an impact when the industry you are monitoring uses your own words as evidence of a problem that they need to address. Luckily, this presentation was at the end of the meeting, and by taking off my name tag, I was able to escape without anybody connecting me to the article. (Somehow I doubt that I will be invited back for future conferences.)

Throughout the meeting, speakers routinely vilified plaintiffs' lawyers and public interest groups as the enemy. In quite ominous tones, defense lawyers constantly over-stated the number of groups and plaintiffs' lawyers even considering litigation, let alone actively engaged in the strategy. Numerous times I found myself stifling smiles and shaking my head at their exaggerated fears. They spoke of hordes of "very well-funded" plaintiffs' lawyers in cahoots with dozens of public interest groups, carefully plotting the avalanche of lawsuits against Big Food. And yet, they seemed oddly at a loss to name specific people, with two or three exceptions, which they just repeated over and over.

I can come up with only two competing explanations for this rift with reality: either the presenters truly believed their words and thus were very misinformed, or the defense attorneys running the conference were deliberately inflating the threat to ensure the need for their expensive services—to help food companies "minimize liability." My cynical nature makes me lean more toward the latter explanation.

Lobbying against phantom threats

The National Restaurant Association (NRA) and the Food

Products Association (FPA, formerly the National Food Processors Association) have been the two key players convincing willing legislators to sponsor legislation to protect industry. At the industry conference, Scott Riehl, FPA's vice president of government affairs, admitted that lobbying for these bills is a deliberate strategy to preempt litigation. In other words, he's fully aware that no *actual* threat of litigation exists. But why let pesky facts get in the way? He gleefully explained how easy it was to get bills enacted because trial lawyers were not mounting significant opposition.

So, you might be wondering, if greedy trial lawyers were truly on the verge of filing an onslaught of obesity-related lawsuits, wouldn't they be engaged in an aggressive counter-lobbying campaign? Of course, since trial lawyers aren't filing obesity-related cases, it makes sense that they wouldn't waste resources opposing these bills. Also, trial lawyers are facing even larger "tort reform" threats to the *actual* types of lawsuits they file, such as medical malpractice. But such reality-based reasoning cannot deter a trade-group lobbyist.

As I sat listening to Riehl proudly rattle off shield-law victories state by state, the real motivation for his group's intense interest dawned on me: self-survival. Because industry trade associations are so costly to join, they must continuously justify their existence to potential and ongoing members. And because lobbying is the main selling point for any trade group, dreaming up new reasons to lobby is a great way to position your services as essential.

Whether the actual policies trade groups lobby for are necessary or even logical is quite beside the point. As long as they have something to show for themselves to keep their deep-pocketed members, trade groups can stay in the game. This self-preservation motivation explains why lobbyists would overstate the threat of litigation: to justify to politicians and the public the need to pass these bills.

Reading off the same sheet of music

The politicians sponsoring these bills are essentially acting as puppets of industry and are taking full advantage of the corporate lobbying. "We've had lots of wonderful support from industry," boasted (federal bill sponsor) Congressman Ric Keller's chief of staff Bryan Malenius. "The National Restaurant Association has done a wonderful job of helping coordinate these state-by-state efforts and we are all reading off the same sheet of music."[12]

Indeed, the NRA works quite effectively in tandem with each state's restaurant association. On a page titled "State Frivolous-Lawsuit Legislation," NRA's Web site tracks the legislative progress in each state.[13] (I use this page myself as a convenient, time-saving way to keep up on the latest developments.) NRA's Web site also offers an entire "Obesity Issue Kit" that includes model legislation, op-ed articles, talking points, and other resources, all designed to assist states in the effort to both pass legislation and to shield industry from liability.[14] So while local politicians try to position these bills as protecting the poor small-restaurant owner, in reality, the policy is backed by strong national forces that represent the food industry's largest companies.

Dismantling the Rhetoric

Industry's high-powered lobbying effort is actually about much more than just passing bills. A convenient side effect of this lobbying crusade is to apply corporate spin to maximum effect. The rhetoric surrounding the lobbying shapes the broader debate related to who is to blame for obesity and diet-related health problems. Because lawsuits are such a hot-button issue, industry can take full advantage of the popular scapegoating of trial lawyers, while at the same time invoke all-American values and shove the personal responsibility theory down the nation's collective throat.

Personal responsibility to the rescue

As discussed earlier, the food industry is fond of pointing to personal responsibility as the "true solution" to the obesity problem. The federal bill's official name, "The Personal Responsibility in Food Consumption Act," says it all. A critical strategy of food companies as they come under increasing attack is to discredit the very idea of litigation in the public's mind long before they even get to the courtroom. That goal is at the heart of applying the "personal responsibility" rhetoric to these bills. If people believe that only individuals are responsible for their own eating behaviors, then companies cannot be blamed for any untoward consequences through litigation.

A lawsuit by definition is frivolous

Another important rhetorical trick is the relentless use of the phrase "frivolous lawsuits." As in: passage of these bills is needed to protect poor mom-and-pop companies from all the frivolous lawsuits being brought by greedy lawyers. This tactic is designed to appeal to those politicians already inclined to attack trial lawyers. Attaching the word *frivolous* to the word *lawsuit* at every opportunity gives the impression that *any* lawsuit filed by a consumer is frivolous, which is an attempt to undermine potential public sympathy for the concept in general.

More subtly, referring specifically to the McDonald's case filed in New York as an example of a "frivolous lawsuit" is a great way to plant the idea in the public's mind that the case is groundless. However, an appeals court judge overturned the trial court's decision to dismiss the case, suggesting that the plaintiff's evidence at the very least deserves to be heard.

As American as cheeseburgers and common sense

No one is really sure how it started, but at some point people started using the nickname "cheeseburger bills" to refer to the proposed shield laws, and the media has gleefully perpetuated this. Invoking the name of a common food that so many people love works wonders for industry. How could we allow lawsuits over anything so American? Various state versions of the bill also use the name "Commonsense Consumption Act." Why, it's good old-fashioned common sense to not sue companies over personal eating habits—who could argue with that? In order to help reframe the issue, I prefer to call the bills "shield laws," because they aim to shield industry from legal liability.

Bill proponents also like to use the image of mom-and-pop businesses at risk of being targeted for legal action. Ellen Fried says that in bill hearings, proponents often trot out the small-restaurant owners who say they are afraid of being sued, but they are really just puppets. "It's been framed as the small-restaurant owners versus the greedy trial lawyers, as opposed to the companies who sell highly processed foods all over the country without identifying what's in the food, versus unsuspecting consumers."[15]

Next, Let's Kill All the Lawyers

In addition to the trade associations, another important player in the effort to shield industry from legal liability is the Center for Consumer Freedon (CCF), the notorious food and restaurant industry front group. (See Chapter 3 for more background.) CCF has assisted the lobbying effort through a multipronged approach that includes congressional testimony, strategic placement of op-ed articles, and extensive advertising campaigns.

CCF clearly recognizes the power of advertising. They have launched numerous campaigns in both print and television, all designed to control the terms of the debate, mainly by attacking trial lawyers for being greedy and unscrupulous.

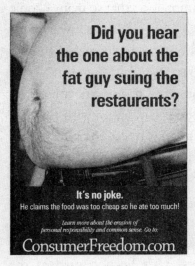

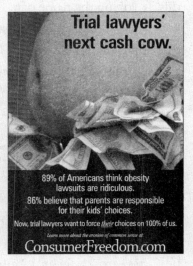

These two CCF print ads make fun of obesity-related lawsuits by accusing lawyers of seeking to get rich off some poor guy's beer belly.

To the question of whether I heard the one about the fat guy suing the restaurants (see ad), I would have to say no, since there is no such lawsuit. (The only case that might fit the description was filed in 2002 and dropped almost immediately.) But the point of the ad is not to convey the truth, but rather to convince people that the idea of filing a food-related lawsuit is absurd. Never mind that the case pending in New York (on behalf of children) is based on McDonald's deceptive marketing practices and not predicated on the company making anyone fat. Why bother with legal theories that require explanation and reasoning when photos of fat stomachs that appeal to emotion and stereotypes are more effective?

CCF is also running a series of television commercials to illustrate how greedy trial lawyers are. This is the text accompanying one of them on their Web site:

> Greedy trial lawyers are plotting their legal assault against restaurants and food providers in an effort to cash in on the nation's expanding waistline. The Center for Consumer Freedom launched this television commercial to warn Americans that these lawyers are desperately looking for ways to make food their next supersized payday.[16]

Pretty strong language, but par for the course for CCF; note the key phrases: "greedy trial lawyers" (according to CCF, this is the only kind) and "legal assault" (no evidence is provided). And why Americans need to be "warned" about such greedy lawyer behavior is unclear. Moreover, if this ad were true, don't you think more than the one lawsuit might be filed? But reality is of no import to CCF.

The potential impact of CCF's campaign can be found in the pages of newspaper articles reporting on state-by-state attempts to pass shield laws. For example, an article about the debate over the California bill quoted the following directly from CCF's Web site as if it were legitimate information contributing to the debate:

> A cabal of fat-cat trial lawyers are poised to launch an onslaught of frivolous lawsuits to cash in on the debate over America's weight. From restaurants and food producers to doctors, schools and even parents, no target is too big or small for these sharks who see dollar signs where the rest of us see dinner.[17]

Once again, no data is offered to back up this absurd claim, just histrionic and vitriolic language—perfectly designed for members of the media who love a good fight. The reporter made no other reference to CCF's involvement in the legislation, suggesting that the Web site attack was all he needed. The media bears much of the blame for inflating the alleged threat of litigation by repeating industry's exaggerated rhetoric without bothering to check the facts.

CCF's goal is to firmly plant the idea in the public's mind that lawyers are unscrupulous and that any attempt to hold industry accountable through the court system is patently absurd. Never mind that only one lawsuit has been filed, that a federal appeals court found that case worthy of consideration, or that the imaginary cabal of greedy lawyers has yet to win a single dime.

California's Puppet Politician Fails to Persuade

Because of my concern that these shield laws could have an adverse impact on consumers, coupled with my contempt for the arrogance and deceit demonstrated by the corporate lobbying, I decided to play a role in fighting the passage of the bill in my home state of California. So I went to the state capital of Sacramento to witness policy making in action. It was not a pretty sight.

In February 2004, California assemblyman John Dutra introduced a bill to shield the food industry from legal liability. It has become painfully obvious to me that politicians are being used as pawns in these corporate lobbying efforts. This is the only explanation for what happened in the state legislative chamber. In his statement in support of the measure to the assembly judiciary committee, Dutra said: "A number of frivolous lawsuits have been filed recently in other states against restaurants and food manufacturers claiming they are responsible for some individuals' overweight and obesity-related health conditions."[18] However, Dutra offered no specific figures or examples. To say that this statement amounts to lying to a legislative body would not be inaccurate. In his defense, Dutra was likely reading from talking points provided by industry. Not that this is any excuse; why aren't the sponsoring lawmaker's staffers checking these "facts"?

He continued: "In my view, these are baseless claims and naive lawsuits and a shameful distraction from finding sensible solutions to the very complex and serious issue of obesity in America. More attention needs to be paid to educating the public on the importance of healthy lifestyles, moderation, and personal responsibility, not more senseless litigation."[19] The rhetoric of "sensible solutions," "complex," "moderation," and "personal responsibility" is all taken directly from industry's playbook, suggesting that the California Restaurant Association or another industry group told Dutra exactly what to say. Moreover, if there was ever a "shameful distraction" from "finding sensible solutions," it's the effort to pass these bills. Instead of passing laws to (for example) get healthier food into schools, legislatures are wasting their time and resources shielding industry from liability. Even though I figured that industry had put Dutra up to it, I was still disgusted that he could get away with spouting such disingenuous rhetoric during a legislative hearing.

Dutra's puppet strings were being pulled by a powerful cadre of food and other probusiness organizations. The opposition consisted of a few small nonprofit nutrition-advocacy organizations, along with one state consumer lawyers' group. At the hearing, only two nutrition advocates testified —myself and Harold Goldstein, director of the California Center for Public Health Advocacy. Despite being outnumbered, we managed to defeat the bill, thanks to a Democrat-controlled legislature that is traditionally friendly to trial lawyers. Industry came back in 2005 to try and pass the bill a second time, again to no avail.

Despite the victory, my colleagues and I diverted our very limited time and resources from other important activities. This is also part of industry's strategy: to keep advocates on the defensive. That way, we will be distracted from concentrating on genuine threats to industry's bottom line, such as getting junk food out of schools and promoting nutrition labeling in restaurants.

Understanding How Lawsuits Work

Because most nutrition advocates act only in support of a bill (and rarely employ lobbyists to hang around state capitols monitoring legislation, as industry does), many states have been caught by surprise, unable to organize collective action in opposition. Knowing a few basic legal concepts will help.

Lawsuits are expensive and risky

Because filing a lawsuit takes such a tremendous amount of resources, few plaintiffs' lawyers are out there filing cases willy-nilly, especially against corporate defendants who can easily outspend them. Most plaintiffs' lawyers are hired on a contingency basis, meaning that they initially work for free, paying all the up-front costs, and then only get paid at the very end if they win the case. These potentially costly risks discourage the filing of "frivolous lawsuits."

Lawsuits are thrown out all the time

Courts already disallow baseless claims through the normal course of legal procedures. Corporate defense lawyers are not helpless and have ample opportunity to ask the court to dismiss baseless cases early on in the litigation process; all lawyers take full advantage of these existing legal rules.

Judges can impose fines on lawyers

In addition, if a lawyer files a case that is later dismissed, the opposing counsel can ask the judge to sanction that lawyer for filing a frivolous claim that wasted time and resources. Lawyers don't like to have to pay fines, so this

rule serves an as additional strong deterrent to filing baseless claims.

Food companies are prolific litigators

Food-industry lawyers file thousands of lawsuits to benefit
corporate interests, some of which even seek to silence
industry critics. For example, the soda industry sued the U.S.
government to keep marketing in public schools. And in
England, McDonald's sued two activists for criticizing the
fast-food chain, resulting in the "McLibel" case and the
longest trial (ten years) in British history.

For a detailed list of counterarguments, see Appendix 5.

What's at Stake

While it's too soon to predict the impact of these bills, I am
concerned about what the future holds. So far, most of the
laws have been passed in states without much consumer litigation activity. (A notable exception is Illinois.) Also, we
don't yet know how broadly the laws will be applied. Federal
bill sponsor Congressman Ric Keller defends the federal
measure by claiming that it is "narrowly drawn." But the
courts will ultimately decide, making it a crapshoot—
depending on which judge makes the call.

It's also possible that many of these bills are unconstitutional, another "minor technicality" that is of no consequence to corporate lobbyists. Most state constitutions
guarantee its citizens access to the court system. But again,
this question will be subject to judicial interpretation,
which means an unpredictable outcome. Once passed, unconstitutional laws can remain on the books until they are

challenged. Meantime, the chilling effect takes hold and the damage is done.

If a federal shield law passes, the implications could be enormous, since it would ban lawsuits in all fifty states as well as federal cases in one fell swoop. Attempting to bar potential litigants from the courthouse is a popular political idea in Washington. The Bush administration is currently engaged in a much broader crusade against the civil justice system. That's why this effort isn't about to go away anytime soon. The rhetoric of "frivolous lawsuits" fits nicely with turning trial lawyers into prominent scapegoats for the nation's economic woes.

This issue also presents a golden opportunity for food-industry lobbyists to fight back while avoiding corporate accountability. Industry's effort to preemptively shield itself from legal liability is hypocritical and disingenuous. If food companies are so worried about becoming targets of lawsuits, why don't they change their business practices to act more responsibly? For starters, restaurants could provide nutrition information for their patrons. Food companies that heavily target young children could reconsider that marketing strategy. Why won't they? Because it costs less to fund a powerful lobbying effort to pass laws that restrict access to the courtroom than it does to clean up your act. Instead of being part of the solution, food companies and their lobbyists are making sure they won't be held accountable for remaining part of the problem.

13

The Bigger Picture

If we don't do the impossible, we shall be faced with the unthinkable.[1]

—Petra Kelly, German politician

I hope it is clear by now: we cannot trust food corporations—not to make healthier food, not to stop marketing to children, and certainly not to help forge meaningful nutrition policy. At every opportunity, corporations place their own profit motives ahead of the public interest. Simply put, the food industry cannot be "part of the solution" to the nation's diet-related health problems.

Where, then, do we go from here? While I do not claim to have all of the answers, I can offer a few modest proposals. In addition to the specific suggestions offered throughout this book, here are some "bigger picture" ideas.

Industry-Laid Traps: Don't Believe the Hype

Because food companies are primarily motivated by the bottom line, all their talk of helping Americans live healthier lives in the end amounts to little more than self-serving PR. The real question is always: who actually benefits from their self-initiated "reforms"? To hear food makers tell it, the "consumer" is the prime beneficiary; but ultimately, corporations have the most to gain. As soon as a policy change begins to undermine a corporation's guiding principle of profit maximization, it's likely to be watered down or revoked entirely at the urging of the chief financial officer. Either way, the public health suffers.

Here, then, are some of the key traps to avoid when considering the next pronouncement from a food corporation.

The media trap

Journalists (whether under the pressure of a tight deadline or out of sheer laziness) too often rely only on corporate sources when reporting complex stories. Therefore, I am often skeptical of media accounts of a company announcement. It's always better to read the original press release—usually available on the company's Web site—for the complete details. Typically, the release is more straightforward and truthful than the press report.

The false security trap

As we've seen, staving off the threat of government regulation and lawsuits is a main objective of many industry policy initiatives. Insisting that their own self-regulatory efforts are on the job, food companies seek to lull policy makers and the general public into a false sense of security. Many experts have been eager to embrace these voluntary moves, thinking that food makers are handing them an easy victory for public health. This is understandable, given the political compromises and uphill battle advocates face when pursuing legislation and other expensive, time-consuming policy strategies. But the real beneficiaries of self-regulation are corporations, which effectively do an end run around the law by promising to abide by their own unenforceable rules.

When a soft drink company, for instance, announces a voluntary policy to remove certain beverages from schools, policy makers and advocates should consider if it's worth trading mandatory legislation for a corporate policy that can and will be rescinded if it poses a threat to quarterly earnings. Of course, legislation is also subject to political wind shifting, but laws are harder to overturn and at least offer viable enforcement mechanisms.

The applause trap

Food companies are masters at turning criticism into marketing opportunities, and at getting us to give them credit for "addressing" problems that they created in the first place. (The recent spate of "trans fat free" marketing is a classic example.) Nutrition advocates who buy into the myth of industry-created solutions do so at their own peril. Praising companies for "doing the right thing" only encourages more food-industry PR (or "nutriwashing"), which in turn results in further mollifying of policy makers and critics. I am not saying that we should stop complaining and let companies off the hook for their excessive marketing practices, especially those that exploit children. But we certainly shouldn't greet corporations that claim to be changing their ways with a warm round of applause. Industry's own well-heeled PR firms are already working overtime to pat food manufacturers on the back. The last thing they need is more cheerleaders.

Also, lauding firms like McDonald's and Kraft for "improving" their products legitimizes the current industrialized food model. Believe it or not, humans once subsisted on food that came exclusively from nature, not a factory. We did not evolve on a diet of Whoppers, Ring Dings, and Orange Crush and will never thrive on lower-salt, lower-fat, or lower-sugar versions of these industrial pseudofoods. We need a more holistic, sustainable strategy that doesn't simply accept the status quo as inevitable (more on this below).

The partnership trap

The idea of "working with" the food industry to solve the nation's diet-related health problems is becoming increasingly attractive to many health experts, nutrition advocates, and policy makers. With surprising enthusiasm, they've entered into various "public-private partnerships" with food sellers, contributing their expertise to health advisory boards and other impressive-sounding bodies. As we've seen, such alliances provide industry with much-needed legitimacy and PR cover but do little to safeguard public health. Meanwhile, what price is society paying from health experts' efforts to "work with industry"?

At the 2004 *Time*/ABC News Summit on Obesity, Kelly Brownell, director of Yale's Rudd Center for Food Policy and

Obesity, was skeptical of food-industry calls for collaboration, noting the lessons learned from tobacco control: "The early days of tobacco history involved everybody standing around the campfire holding hands and saying we need to collaborate, cooperate. We paid a huge price for that because it stalled public health efforts to control tobacco for decades, and who knows how many millions of people died as a consequence."[2]

We are now facing a similar situation with the food industry. Northeastern law professor Richard Daynard agrees that nutrition advocates would do well to remember the lessons learned in the fight against cigarette makers. Industry's goals, he insists, are "antithetical to public health," making the notion of partnering with them "absurd." Daynard explains that:

> [y]ou can't partner with someone who has a totally different set of goals than you. You may be able to reach a truce, or cut a deal if you have something to threaten them with. Then you can get them to stop behaving as badly as they otherwise would have. But the situation is hopeless unless you go into it with the understanding that your interests are almost diametrically opposed, and that any deal you reach will be with an adversary.[3]

Health experts and others currently partnering with industry will be sadly disappointed if they believe that significant changes will result. In the meantime, we all pay the price as more promising reform strategies and movement-building efforts are passed over. How long will it take until we realize that industry is not on our side?

Getting caught unprepared: take the lobbying seriously

In this book, we've seen a number of examples of local campaigns that have faced powerful counterassaults from Big Food. These valiant efforts show the importance of shoring up resources to take on one of the most well-funded corporate lobbying machines in the nation. As Representative Sean Faircloth of Maine observes, public health advocates need to be ready to step up to the plate, just as they did with Big Tobacco. He says you have to go in "knowing that you are always going to be outgunned. That's just the reality; but you've got to bring a gun. You can't just have volunteers come in, once or twice. They do a good job; I don't mean to belittle them, but this cannot be done part-time. This requires a full-force lobbying effort."[4]

Many health and nutrition groups are used to conducting relatively neutral, uncontentious educational campaigns. It's time for such organizations (including funders) to shift more resources to advocacy and make policy efforts a higher priority, and not shy away from controversy. Educational efforts are futile without strong policies in place to support people's ability to make healthy food choices.

The Obesity Trap:
Shifting the Focus to Causes, Not Symptoms

In 1996, I began working in the area of nutrition advocacy. Then all of a sudden, in 2002, just after the release of "The Surgeon General's Call to Action to Prevent and Decrease Overweight and Obesity," I found myself working on "obesity." While I am grateful for the many dedicated public health advocates who have joined the "fight against obesity," I find this trend problematic on a number of levels. I understand that focusing on obesity makes sense in certain medical contexts—for example, with people who suffer from obesity-related health problems such as diabetes. (Although many people develop diet-related health problems without becoming obese.) However, I'm concerned that recent efforts to frame nutrition policy around obesity are shortsighted and ultimately best serve the interests of the food industry.

If you think about it, obesity is only one *symptom* of a much larger, underlying problem: a profit-driven, corporate-controlled food supply. We should devote our energies to fixing the root problem (the food system) rather than squander our precious resources on symptoms like obesity. Notice that advocates working to reduce smoking rates are in the field of "tobacco control," not "lung cancer" or "emphysema." (Among the few exceptions are the American Lung Association and American Cancer Society, but these are organizations that mainly prefer to play it safe politically.) Just as lung cancer is *one* result of smoking (a bad habit encouraged by the savvy marketing strategies of the tobacco industry), obesity is *one* result of poor diet (another bad habit fostered by the equally manipulative marketing practices of the food industry).

Fueling personal responsibility

Like other distractions, the obesity focus diverts attention away from larger policy questions and dumps the task of solving diet-related health problems squarely in the lap of the individual. Framing obesity as a strictly individual or "lifestyle" problem fits perfectly with industry's "personal responsibility" mantra. Tobacco control advocates were once similarly focused on educating people about the health risks of smoking. But then they realized that broader policy changes such as indoor smoking bans and controls on tobacco companies' marketing practices were critical. Nutrition advocates need to undergo a similar awakening: we must acknowledge the importance of forging policy solutions that hold the food industry responsible for obesity, along with a host of other social ills.

Fueling prejudice and weight-loss obsession

Another problem with the obesity focus is that it serves to reinforce and perpetuate the prejudices that many Americans have against overweight people. What's the first thing you think of when you hear the word *obesity*? A fat person, right? And what stereotypes and biases go along with that? Among other negative traits, obese people are often viewed as lazy and irresponsible, with no one but themselves to blame. Obese people are already subjected to rampant discrimination, for example, in the workplace and health-care settings. The last thing we need is for nutrition advocates to fuel this fire. We also shouldn't perpetuate America's weight-loss obsession—thanks in large part to the $50-billion-a-year industry that caters to this mania. Weight-loss outfits like Weight Watchers keep people hooked on contrived "calorie-restriction" regimens rather than healthful diets, promoting dangerous "weight cycling" (rapidly losing and gaining weight). This can actually be more risky than remaining overweight. Let's not stoke these flames by giving obesity more emphasis than it is due.

Short-lived media attention

It may be true, as a colleague once reminded me, that when we talked about "nutrition," we hardly got any media attention, but now that the focus is "obesity," we're finally on the map. Certainly much of the extensive media coverage over the past several years has had positive ripple effects, such as raising awareness about the importance of good nutrition. But the attention is likely to be short-lived, given that our media is driven by what sells—emotional personal stories and new (often manufactured) controversies. The novelty and "drama" of obesity as a major public health crisis will likely wear thin over time. Remember all of the media devoted to tobacco-related stories in years past? These days such focus is relatively rare, despite the fact that smoking is still by far the number-one cause of preventable death in the United States. Do we really want to base our long-term hopes and strategies on the media's willingness to pay attention to our concerns? We need to be leaders in framing nutrition-policy issues, not followers.

Special implications for children

When tackling the issue of childhood obesity, advocates have identified prevention as a key concern. This is understandable, considering that avoiding excessive weight gain early in life is crucial to forestalling a lifetime of diet-related illness. But with children—no less than with adults—honing in on a symptom like obesity runs the risk of distracting us from other, bigger-picture problems, such as the excessive commercialism and exploitative marketing practices to which kids are now routinely exposed. In her book *Born to Buy*, Boston College sociology professor Juliet Schor demonstrates how our contemporary "junk culture" impacts children's overall well-being. Kids exposed to high levels of commercialism, she notes, tend to be more depressed and anxious, and suffer from lower self-esteem, headaches, stomachaches, and boredom.[5] If we remain fixated on "obesity-related" concerns like the number of calories in soda, we're likely to overlook such broader societal problems affecting children.

Physical activity and nutrition: seperate issues?

These days, the issues of "nutrition" and "physical activity" are often needlessly linked. Sometimes, we're even asked to choose sides. At a conference on childhood obesity, I once observed an audience member express dismay that "her issue," physical activity, was taking a backseat to nutrition—as if the two camps were in competition. Many advocates are perpetuating this problem by insisting that we discuss both "nutrition and physical activity." While they are each vitally important to good health, so are many other lifestyle issues, such as getting enough rest, good dental hygiene, and drinking clean water.

As we've seen, leaders in government and industry love to point to exercise as the real answer to obesity, explaining the problem away as simply a matter of balancing "calories in" (diet) and "calories out" (exercise). Advocacy efforts that focus on obesity also fuel the lack-of-exercise excuse. We shouldn't be muddying up the already extremely complex waters of nutrition policy with that of physical activity. Let's keep the issues separate.

I prefer to avoid the term *obesity* altogether. Instead, I talk about "diet-related public health problems" or simply "nutrition advocacy." "Marketing diseases," a phrase used by the nonprofit Commercial Alert, is another phrase I like, since it also encompasses a broad range of health problems for which the food, tobacco, and alcohol industries are chiefly responsible.

The American Policymaking Trap: Don't Ignore Globalization

We Americans tend to be very egocentric in our thinking about policy making. But in an era of economic and political globalization, confining our strategy to U.S. borders makes little sense. Corporations must continue to grow or they will die. The only place left to go after companies have saturated the U.S. market is abroad. Even if we could somehow "ban" domestic sales of junk food, food corporations would simply carve out new markets overseas—as tobacco sellers have been doing for years. Thanks in part to tobacco-control initiatives here, the United States now makes up only 4 percent of the global tobacco market.[6]

There are already clear signs that U.S.-based food makers are gearing up to follow in Big Tobacco's globalizing footsteps. Developing countries are especially fertile ground for American-style fast-food expansion. China is now home to 800 KFC franchises and 100 Pizza Hut outlets. Yum Brands, the parent company of these chains, brags that China is its "number-one market for new company restaurant development worldwide" and that operating profits there were more than $200 million in 2005.[7] India's fast-food industry is not far behind China's. Growing by 40 percent a year, it's expected to generate over a billion dollars in annual sales—even as a quarter of that nation's population remains undernourished.[8]

We can't talk about globalization without mentioning McDonald's, the company that has come to symbolize American food abroad. Currently boasting more than 30,000 outlets in 119 countries, McDonald's already earns (along with KFC) the majority of its profits outside the United States. Classes at McDonald's Hamburger University are taught in twenty different languages. McDonald's currently has 730 outlets in China and plans to reach 1,000 by 2008.[9] Riding on McDonald's coattails is another American icon, Coca-Cola, whose soft drinks are sold at Golden Arches outlets worldwide. Coke's brands (almost four hundred of them) are now available in more than two hundred countries, and more than 70 percent of the company's income originates outside the United States.[10] Rival PepsiCo is investing an additional $500 million in India alone and hopes to triple its revenues there by 2008.[11] Processed-food giants such as Kraft and General Mills also have plans to globalize their operations.

One of the more insidious ways that American food corporations infiltrate foreign markets is by tailoring their brand marketing to "target local tastes." For example, in China, PepsiCo has concocted Lay's potato chips in flavors such as Hangzhou Stewed Meat and Hokkaido Crab.[12] By invoking these familiar-sounding names, U.S.-based food sellers hope to convince new consumers to abandon their traditional diets in favor of modern, industrialized ones. As an advertising executive in China said with shocking frankness: people must be made to understand that "imported equals good, local equals *crap*." A former president of McDonald's Japan appallingly claimed that "the reason Japanese people are so short and have yellow skin is because they have eaten nothing but rice and fish for two thousand years . . . [I]f we eat McDonald's hamburgers and potatoes for a thousand years, we will become taller, our skin white, and our hair blond."[13]

Far from producing new populations of Westernized "supermen," the exportation of the United States' highly processed, meat-centered diet is having disastrous public health consequences for the developing world, where obesity is spreading. Paradoxically, countries such as India, which continue to be plagued by hunger, are now also suffering from chronic, diet-related diseases that were relatively unknown prior to the invasion of Western-style foods. With this in mind, we must consider the health impacts of the industrial food system as worldwide problems, rather than mainly American or "first world" ones. And we must confront them on a global level; adopting a narrow-minded NIMBY approach to policymaking is both unethical and untenable. Indeed, as public health advocates, it's our responsibility to stop focusing on localized solutions and start addressing underlying structural causes.

The Limitations of Symptom-Based Policymaking

Ultimately, all of the policy strategies discussed in this book boil down to piecemeal, short-term solutions. A campaign aimed at removing soda from school vending machines or trans fat from french fries, for instance, attacks a *symptom* while failing to treat the *disease*. We must confront the powerful forces that control our modern food system head-on. Improving school food is a good place to start, but it's only one place. Without a long-term vision of the ultimate goal and how we might get there, we will just keep putting out fires.

Enormous resources expended

A major problem with the piecemeal policy approach is the enormous resources it takes to wage each battle against corporate lobbying. Despite impressive and courageous efforts, the deck is always stacked against advocates in favor of corporations, which have the cash to send career lobbyists to Washington, D.C. and every state capitol to protect food makers' bottom lines. Consider the recent efforts to reform California's school nutrition policy. After six years of hard work and spending many precious resources, the California legislature in 2005 finally enacted a compromised statewide school nutrition policy—which, incidentally, has yet to be fully implemented. This scenario is being repeated in states all over the nation, and in some places, the fight is just beginning. While such efforts are laudable and we should continue to pursue them, at some point, we have to ask the hard question: is pouring a considerable amount of our energy and money into a protracted campaign to curb in-school sales of unhealthy food and beverages in one state really worth it?

We need to think long and hard about such questions, especially considering how adept corporations are at undermining even the limited legislative victories we occasionally manage to win. If we pass a measure to remove soda from schools today, companies can simply step up their marketing outside school tomorrow. If we restrict junk food sales in one locality tomorrow, companies can ratchet up their marketing efforts in another city, state, or country the next day. I am not saying we should allow schools to sell junk food or that enacting specific or localized legislation is useless. But to move toward a more sustainable, better-nourished world, we'll also need to engage in broader, long-term strategies aimed at attacking the problem at its roots.

The politics of compromise

What you can get is limited by what you ask for. We never get the "moon" quite simply because we never dare to demand it. I asked several school-based nutrition advocates: if they could choose, what result would they really want? All of them said that getting vending machines out of schools altogether would be best. Why? Because they believe that this is the right, moral, and just thing to do. They also tell me they fear that companies cannot be trusted to abide by rules, so it's better to get rid of them altogether. They know in their hearts that corporations don't belong in schools, and that schools should be a safe haven for children. And yet, sadly, these advocates don't feel that they can speak up for this position publicly. To do so, they fear, would mean being marginalized, exiled from the community of more "reasonable" advocates, where they would no longer be able to accomplish anything. When you're afraid of getting nothing, then compromising—exempting high schools from soda restrictions, for example—begins to look like a good option. But why do we accept such bargaining and political wheeling and dealing over such important matters as children's health as an inevitable part of our political process? Why can't these advocates speak up?

It's not as if we haven't given these strategies a good enough shot. We tend to forget history and think that we are the first generation of advocates to "discover" that kids are being marketed to, when experts have been complaining about this problem for at least thirty years. In the 1970s, the main concern was sugar-related dental problems. Today childhood obesity is the "hot" issue. But whatever the focus, advocates continue to attack the symptoms, rather than take on the underlying cause of the entire public health mess: an unjust and broken food system. Meanwhile, the situation has only gotten worse. If the current approach isn't working, maybe it's time for a new, bolder strategy.

Toward a Broader Vision: Linking Movements

Now for some good news: there are currently a number of social and political movements under way that are questioning the current food system and are offering viable and environmentally sound alternatives. These efforts go by different names, including sustainable agriculture, community food security, food justice, and various "buy local" campaigns. These movements are united in their desire to create more holistic alternatives to the present food system, and provide all people with access to healthy, locally grown food.

Sustainable agriculture advocates, for example, do not see McDonald's salads as the answer. Instead, they promote alternative food systems based on organic and sustainable farming practices designed to preserve the ecology. Such inspiring efforts include farmers' markets, community-supported agriculture (buying shares in a local farm), community gardens, and independent stores and co-ops, to name just a few. One of my favorite programs is called "farm-to-school," through which local farmers supply school lunch programs with fresh, healthful produce. There are hundreds of such alternative movements throughout the country, and their numbers are growing. Working at the community, state, and national levels, they are refusing to accept the current corporate-controlled food system. Instead, they are proposing creative alternatives and making their visions a reality.

While some nutrition advocates are linking arms with these movements, we need to create many more cross linkages. But both groups still need a longer-term vision. Many of these movements believe that we can simply "opt out" of the current industrial food economy, naively thinking that a few farmers' markets and community gardens are going to save us from the likes of Kraft and McDonald's. The fact remains, however, that these corporate behemoths and the political system that sustains them aren't going away unless and until we confront them head-on. As one commentator on the sustainable agriculture movement notes:

> To begin moving our food system in a more just, sustainable, and humane direction, activists must broaden the terms and parameters of the current food policy discourse. They must begin to talk about dismantling the mechanisms of corporate rule—about taking the what, how, and why of food production out of the hands of private, self-interested food producers and giving it to communities and institutions that could democratically determine how to produce and distribute food. Local community-garden and food-security movements are important steps in this direction, as are efforts to contest the "personhood" rights of corporations and global "free-trade" initiatives . . . Buoyed

by the strength of their collective numbers, [activists] could begin to construct an incrementalist reform agenda that is ever mindful of the idea that another world is possible.[14]

We cannot allow a small group of private corporations to continue to dictate the food and nutrition policies of the nation and indeed the world. The crucial question is: who should have the power to make decisions about how we live?

Starting with the Right Questions

Many books like this one conclude with a neat little checklist of "things you can do." Some books critical of the food system often advise you to "vote with your fork" and recommend a list of specific foods to eat to make the world a healthier place. I won't do that. I can tell you that I have chosen to eat a mostly organic, whole-food (unprocessed), plant-based diet as a way of making my own political statement. I also believe that eating this way is optimum for my health, as well as that of the planet, and results in the least harm to animals and workers—all values that resonate with me. (And I happen to enjoy how I eat immensely.) But I also recognize that most people lack access to affordable and sustainable alternatives to industrialized food. The sad fact is that the way I eat is beyond the reach of much of the world's population. That's why we cannot improve the global situation one politically correct forkful at a time. Rather, we must make a fundamental shift in how as a society we produce, transport, market, and sell food—both in this country and around the world—and create viable policies and institutions to support such changes.

As much as I'd like to, I can't provide you with a list of key laws to pass, a twelve-step program to follow, or a "dream team" of attorneys capable of bringing about such a major social and economic transformation. That I don't profess to have a blueprint for how to change the world will likely be frustrating to many readers.

But it's really not up to me to provide the answers. Creating a better world must be a truly democratic process, arising out of grassroots movements, in which the people whose lives are most impacted are included in the decision-making process. What I can do instead is offer you a perspective on the current food system that you're not likely to find elsewhere. I can offer you the reasons why, as I have throughout this book, current reform strategies aren't working, and why we cannot continue to work within a broken system. Armed with these insights, we can work together to find solutions. So while I don't claim to have all of the answers, here are some questions I think we should be asking.

Where do we begin?

First and foremost, we have to change the way we frame food-policy issues. We must challenge the "conventional wisdom"—for example, that children will eat better if we just put SpongeBob images on bags of spinach or if we invest more money in nutrition education programs like "5 a Day." Rather than fall back on these symptom-based "solutions," we need to start an honest discussion about how we got here in the first place.

Next, we must rethink and reprioritize our key concerns. If small battles like removing sodas from schools remain our top priority, we can only hope to win small victories. But if we shift our focus to bigger-picture problems like the commercialization of childhood or the corporate takeover of the food supply, then our demands and goals will be more far-reaching and substantive.

What is the underlying cause of the problem?

Over the last century, the human diet has been radically altered. The foods we eat now bear little resemblance to those that sustained our ancestors for millennia. In their ceaseless pursuit of profits and new markets, a small number of multinational corporations are running roughshod across the globe in flagrant disregard for public health, the environment, and the welfare of workers and farm animals. We have to stop dancing around the issue and admit this simple truth. In recent years, the privatization of water has spurred global activists to mount passionate and inspiring campaigns against the takeover of another substance essential to human survival. Why aren't those of us concerned with food raising similar demands? Like water (and unlike most other commodities such as toys or electronics), food is indispensable and a basic human right. Why have we turned its production over to private interests? Shouldn't at least some aspects of society remain off-limits to corporate control?

Why don't we ask "should" questions?

We must begin to ask "should" questions rather than simply settle for crumbs left over from political compromises. What *should* we be feeding our kids? *Shouldn't* we have clean water fountains in every school? What *should* our food system look like? What's the just and moral outcome? We won't have many opportunities to raise such difficult questions if we only aim to utilize avenues like legislation or litigation—tools that don't readily lend themselves to serious moral or ethical reflection. But how will we ever create a truly better world unless we first figure out what that should be?

Where do we go from here?

We need to take a giant step back and ask, what kind of world do we want to live in? Instead of asking how we can tweak the current lousy system and make it marginally better, let's ask how we can create an entirely new system.

If we could start from scratch and create a truly just food system, what attributes would we want? I might say: sustainable, affordable, accessible, and convenient. You might have other ideas. We need to begin discussing and debating this crucial question now, democratically and openly—in the media, in our schools, in our community centers, everywhere and anywhere we can.

But, you might ask, isn't the idea of taking on the whole system simply too overwhelming? Yes, it is completely overwhelming and it makes me want to run back to bed and pull the covers over my head. Some will say I am being unrealistic because what I am asking will require a major social movement—or maybe many movements working together. That's a formidable goal, yes, but what is the alternative? More symptom-based solutions that do not address the underlying problem? While it certainly seems daunting, I just don't see any alternative if our hope is to create lasting and meaningful social change.

So, how and where can we start to open up this new conversation? Here are a few suggestions for how to get these ideas out into the public discourse:

- The media: write op-ed articles and letters to the editor to your local newspaper about the problems related to the current food system.
- Newsletters: if your organization has a nutrition newsletter, put that "recipe of the month" column on the back burner and run a feature story on nutrition policy and the corporate control of the food supply.
- Conferences: these days, "obesity" conferences are becoming more popular. If you plan to attend such a meeting, request that the organizers broaden the agenda from the usual individual behavior-change model to the public health problems created by an industrial food system and alternatives to it (e.g., farmers' markets and community-based agriculture).
- Workplace: host lunchtime discussions with your colleagues about the effects of the present food system on diet and health. Discuss alternatives.
- Houses of worship, community centers: host talks at your local church or social group about community-based challenges to healthy eating.
- Look for any opportunity to broaden the discussion about food and nutrition to include an open debate about the underlying causes.
- See Appendix 6 for a list of groups and resources to help you get involved.

The current food system is broken and cannot be fixed without a major overhaul. Some may think I am painting a depressing picture, but what could be more hopeful than insisting that another world is possible? We have to start talking about the concerns raised in this book in a whole new way. People need food to survive and thrive; it's a matter of social justice. These are deeply moral issues and addressing them is a complex matter with no pat solutions. But if we are truly committed to putting people before profits, we have to start somewhere.

Appendix 1

ANTI-GLOSSARY

Understanding corporate-speak is a powerful tool for getting at the truth. Once you realize that corporations have very calculated ways of describing their practices, you can begin to see right through the PR spin. Here are just some examples of the lingo.

Activist judges: Any judge who has the potential to rule against a food company in a consumer lawsuit. As in: "We have to pass laws to ban obesity-related lawsuits because we cannot trust activist judges to throw the case out." But in reality, most judges are quite conservative and do not often rule against corporate interests.

Advergaming: Web-based games commonly used to promote junk food to children. Web sites include Postopia.com and NabiscoWorld.com, both owned by Kraft.

Astroturf campaign: Refers to seemingly grassroots groups or coalitions that are actually fake, often created by corporations or public relations firms.

Balanced diet: The oversimplified and meaningless way that food companies like to describe how to eat. The purpose is to keep people confused about nutrition while maintaining the status quo. As in, "All foods can fit into a balanced diet."

Better-for-you products: Processed-food companies' way of describing self-defined nutritionally "superior" foods, using their worst product as comparison. For example, PepsiCo describes its Baked Lays chips as "better for you" than regular fried chips.

Brand loyalty: The tendency of consumers to continue buying a specific brand's product or service despite the competition. Food companies fiercely compete for brand loyalty, which results in ubiquitous marketing.

Branding: The process whereby brand image is developed to make consumers think there is something special about one cola, hamburger, etc., over another.

Buzz or viral marketing: Tactics designed to get people to talk about (create a buzz) or pass along messages about a brand or product. It's especially popular for corporations to aim this technique at teenagers.

Callouts (aka flags): Marketing technique on food packaging to indicate some dubious health benefit. For example, "trans fat free" or "Sensible Solution."

Character merchandising: Employing the use of popular fictional characters to market products to children. Most ubiquitous example: SpongeBob SquarePants.

Cheeseburger bills: The nickname given (by either the media or industry) to bills being passed by a number of states that would bar consumers from suing food companies, the scope of which remain unclear. Inspired by a lawsuit filed against McDonald's.

Choice (aka options): How food lobbyists like to justify maintaining the status quo and deflect government regulation. As in: "We are providing Americans with a wide array of food choices." But we should ask who gets to decide what those "choices" are.

Cobranding: When two companies form a new product together, such as Reese's Puffs cereal (Hershey and General Mills).

Commitment: The tired word used by food companies and trade associations to position themselves as "part of the solution." As in: "We are making a number of commitments to do our part in solving obesity."

Communicate: Corporate marketing euphemism for advertising. As in: "We rely on a number of ways to communicate the benefits of our products to consumers."

Complex issue: How industry selectively describes obesity. For example, in talking about regulating junk food sales in schools, companies argue that it won't work because obesity is such a complex issue. Curiously, though, the problem becomes less complex when the proposed solution is personal responsibility or exercise.

Convenience: The way that industry describes most highly processed, packaged foods, to give the impression that they are helpful to the consumer. But we should ask: convenient for whom?

Corporate responsibility: Another way that Big Food proclaims itself as part of the solution. As in: "Corporate responsibility is part of our DNA" (McDonald's). Also, many companies have annual corporate-responsibility reports that now include alleged "commitments" to reducing obesity.

Cross-promotion: A sales promotion technique whereby the advertisement or promotion for one product includes a promotional message for another product; for example, *Star Wars* toys at Burger King.

Energy balance: The oversimplified term that food executives use to explain obesity in a way that sounds objective and scientific, but which conveniently obscures overconsumption of their unhealthy products. It also has the added benefit of emphasizing weight loss and physical activity, keeping the focus on individual behavioral change.

Exclusive contracting/pouring rights: When soda companies (mainly Coca-Cola and PepsiCo) form contracts with schools to have the right to sell only that company's products on school grounds. Often these deals last for many years, and can contain lucrative signing bonuses and incentives that result in promoting unhealthy beverages.

Food nazi aka food police/cops: How some lobbyists like to refer to nutrition advocates who dare to call on the government to enact reasonable regulations.

Free speech: Guaranteed by the First Amendment and invoked by food lobbyists to justify the status quo related to out-of-control marketing of junk food, especially to kids. But there is no absolute right to free speech, especially for corporations.

Freedom: What some food lobbyists invoke (along with choice) to play on American values and strike fear into the hearts of Americans. As in: "The food police are trying to take away your freedom to enjoy Big Macs and milkshakes."

Frivolous lawsuits: The right wing's favorite moniker for any lawsuit filed by a consumer against a corporate interest. Food lobbyists have adopted it to describe the imaginary onslaught of obesity-related lawsuits against food companies.

Fun-for-you products: Foods with no nutritional benefit, as described by companies like PepsiCo seeking to distinguish its other "better-for-you products." Of course, it wouldn't be so great for sales to call them "bad-for-you."

Functional benefit: How food marketers like to describe certain unhealthy products, such as sports drinks, claiming they provide "energy" or "hydration."

Good or bad foods: As in: "There are no good or bad foods; all foods can fit into a balanced diet." This is how food companies (and many nutritionists who perpetuate this myth) keep people confused and deflect any criticism about unhealthy products.

Good-for-you products: How PepsiCo defines that subsection of its Smart Spot products that they say are "actively good for you," such as Tropicana orange juice or Quaker oatmeal. This is to distinguish from (and place on a higher plane than) the "better-for-you" products such as Diet Pepsi and Baked Lays. (See "better-for-you.")

Government relations/affairs: Industry's euphemism for lobbying. A corporate executive with a title such as "vice president, government relations" is probably a lobbyist.

Halo effect: Forming an overall positive impression because of one good characteristic. For example, McDonald's seeks to earn a halo effect for promoting salads since a belief that the company is now selling healthier food might draw consumers in.

Healthy lifestyles: Another way of distracting attention away from talking about food. As in: "We believe, as do many nutrition experts, that solving the obesity problem is about maintaining a healthy lifestyle and achieving the proper energy balance" (Grocery Manufacturers Association).

Heavy users: Loosely defined as the 20 percent of fast-food eaters who account for 60 percent of all fast-food sales. A typical heavy user is male, in his twenties or thirties and extremely loyal to burgers and fries—where fast-food companies make most of their money.

Host selling: Where a character appearing in a television show also appears in a commercial during that show. This is illegal for children's television, but there are numerous workarounds.

Hydration: Makers of "sports drinks" such as Gatorade claim their products offer "hydration" benefits and that such products "hydrate better than water." But most sports drinks are full of sugar and much of the research is conducted on marathon athletes.

In-store promotions: A catchall term for the wide variety of sales promotions and advertisement efforts that occur at the point of purchase. For example, kids are lured into fast-food outlets with toy promotions.

Initiative: Self-aggrandizing term food companies like to use to describe any excuse for a press release. The idea is to position themselves as "part of the solution" by announcing some great new "initiative" such as an educational program for schools.

Interactive product placement: Planned marketing technology to enable viewers to instantly purchase products used by characters they see in movies and TV programs.

Junk science: The generalized term the right wing uses to describe any science that goes against corporate interests. For example, bona fide research that soda is linked to obesity is often dismissed by soda-industry lobbyists as "junk science."

Licensing: When owners of certain copyrights sell their rights to other companies. For example, when Disney sells a license to McDonald's to market movie-related toys.

Local control: The excuse used by multinational companies such as Coca-Cola for why it opposes state legislation to get soda out of schools. If you hear the argument for local control, ask who is making the argument and what interests they represent.

Moderation: How food companies (and many nutritionists) recommend we eat. As in, "Eat all foods in moderation." It's a meaningless word that leaves people in the dark.

Moms: The condescending and sexist way that food companies like to refer to mothers when talking about marketing to children. As in, "We want to help moms make good choices" (paraphrasing PepsiCo). McDonald's even has a "Global Moms Panel."

Nag factor: How marketers refer to the influence that children have on their parents; i.e., to get kids to nag their parents to buy them the junk food they see advertised.

Opportunity: What food companies like to call obesity; as in, "We think this is a great opportunity," meaning they can make money promoting allegedly healthier food.

Parental responsibility: Term food lobbyists use to deflect blame for excessive marketing to children by blaming it all on the parents.

Part of the solution: Food companies claim they are part of the solution to obesity, for example, by marketing healthier products and promoting health education in schools.

Personal responsibility: The concept food lobbyists like to use to deflect criticism by blaming individuals for their fate—never mind the billions of dollars they spend in marketing each year.

Point of purchase: How marketers refer to the placement of certain messages targeting consumers at the moment they make a decision about buying a product to encourage what industry calls "impulse purchases." For example, product packaging blazoned with cartoon characters and placed at a child's eye level at the point of purchase is a critical marketing tool to get young consumers to nag their parents.

Portfolio: How the large food companies refer to their array of brands. As in, "We have a wide portfolio of products that consumers can choose from to meet their needs."

Portion control: Almost every processed-food company now makes 100-calorie "portion control" products, from cookies to popcorn to soda. It's a great way to make you pay more for less while destroying the environment with excessive packaging.

Positives: How some companies like to refer to artificially adding nutrients, such as vitamins, to otherwise unhealthy products. As in, "Our focus has been on reducing fat, reducing sugar, and adding positives" (PepsiCo).

Presweetened: Euphemism for any food that contains a lot of sugar. Mostly used by General Mills to describe its children's cereals to deflect critics. As in, "Even presweetened cereals are the best breakfast your child could eat."

Product placement: When a product appears in a TV program or movie, paid for by the manufacturer to gain exposure.

Public–private partnership: An increasingly common arrangement whereby a government agency or nonprofit organization partners with a food corporation, usually for some health-related promotional activity that focuses on individual behavior change.

Reformulation: One of the strategies processed-food companies are using to trick us into thinking they are making healthier products. For example, General Mills has "reformulated" all of its cereals to contain "whole grain"—even sugary kids' brands.

Self-regulation: The voluntary system of oversight that food corporations prefer to having government meddling in their business practices.

Sensible Solutions: Kraft Foods' self-defined nutritional seal program. Sensible Solutions products marketed to kids include "1\2 the Sugar Fruity Pebbles" and "Pepperoni Flavored Sausage Pizza Lunchables."

Silver bullet: Term food lobbyists like to use to dismiss any regulation that singles out their products. As in: "Getting junk food out of schools is no silver bullet solution to obesity."

Smart Spot: PepsiCo's self-defined nutritional seal program. Smart Spot products include Diet Pepsi, Gatorade, and Baked Lays.

Sound science: The objective-sounding way that food companies like to justify their opposition to any policy that would interfere with their bottom line. As in: "We cannot act to remove soda and junk food from schools in the absence of 'sound science.' " But for industry, no amount of science will ever be sufficient.

Stealth marketing: A technique whereby consumers are not aware that they are being marketed to. Children are especially vulnerable, for example, to product placement.

Suggestive selling: When the clerk or waiter suggests additional food items; restaurants train personnel in this tactic. As in, "Do you want fries with that?"

Third-party experts: When food lobbyists want to hide the biased nature of their scientific conclusions, they often hire third-party experts who have no obvious connection to industry. These experts may testify against nutrition legislation, publish scientific articles, or otherwise represent corporate views without revealing their backing.

Tort reform: What the right wing calls legislation to restrict consumers' access to the courtroom. Laws being passed to ban obesity lawsuits are one example.

Trial lawyers (as in "greedy"): The scapegoat for the nation's economic problems. In the food context, "greedy trial lawyers" are allegedly targeting food makers with "frivolous lawsuits" despite only *one* obesity-related case having been filed so far.

GUIDE TO INDUSTRY GROUPS AND SPIN DOCTORING

The food industry employs many tools to help them lobby and control the nutrition debate. Understanding who the major players are is critical to recognizing them when they appear in the press and to exposing their biases.

Types of groups/programs:
- Trade associations lobby on behalf of their members
- Front groups also lobby, but often hide their corporate backing
- Scientific institutes give the appearance of legitimate research
- Educational programs usually emphasize physical activity as the "solution"
- Public–private partnerships co-opt government and nonprofit groups

Industry Trade Associations—Food and Beverage

American Beverage Association
Represents soft drink companies; formerly called the National Soft Drink Association. Local bottlers are also represented by regional trade groups.
www.ameribev.org

Food Products Association
Represents food and beverage companies; focuses on science and food safety.
www.fpa-food.org

Grocery Manufacturers Association (previously the Grocery Manufacturers of America)
Represents food, beverage, and other "consumer packaged goods" companies that account for $680 billion in annual sales. (Note: FPA and GMA plan to merge as of January 2007, creating an even more powerful lobbying force.)
www.gmabrands.com

National Automatic Merchandising Association
Represents interests of food and beverage vendors and food-service operators.
www.vending.org

National Restaurant Association
Represents 60,000 member companies with more than 300,000 outlets.
www.restaurant.org

Snack Food Association
Represents 800 companies, snack makers, and suppliers worldwide.
www.sfa.org

Industry Trade Associations—Advertising

Alliance for American Advertising
This loosely affiliated group, which includes Kraft Foods, PepsiCo, Kellogg, and General Mills, was formed to defend their "right" to advertise to children.
(No Web site.)

American Advertising Federation
Represents 50,000 professionals and 130 corporate members (advertisers, agencies, and media companies) that comprise the nation's leading brands.
www.aaf.org

American Association of Advertising Agencies
Represents 80 percent of the advertising volume placed by agencies.
www.aaaa.org

Association of National Advertisers
Represents a wide array of corporations to protect "commercial free speech."
www.ana.net

Children's Advertising Review Unit
Industry self-appointed self-regulatory body.
www.caru.org

Industry Trade Associations—Legal

American Legislative Exchange Council
Represents corporate interests, especially in state legislatures.
www.alec.org

American Tort Reform Association
Represents corporations to undermine consumer rights.
www.atra.org

Washington Legal Foundation
Represents corporations through litigation and public relations.
www.wlf.org

Industry Front Groups

American Council on Fitness and Nutrition
Backed by almost every major food corporation.
www.acfn.org

American Council on Science and Health
Backed by an array of corporations to promote industry interests.
www.acsh.org

Center for Consumer Freedom
Backed mainly by the restaurant industry.
www.consumerfreedom.com

Council for Corporate and School Partnerships
Founded by Coca-Cola to further school soda contracts.
www.corpschoolpartners.org

International Food Information Council
Runs Kidnetic.com, among other corporate-friendly programs.
www.ific.org

Whole Grains Council
Provides processed-food makers with a self-defined "stamp" of
approval.
www.wholegrainscouncil.org

Industry Science Institutes and Advisory Boards

The Bell Institute of Health and Nutrition (General Mills)
www.bellinstitute.com

The Beverage Institute for Health and Wellness (Coca-Cola)
www.thebeverageinstitute.org

Blue Ribbon Advisory Board (PepsiCo)
www.smartspot.com/5_commitment/5-3-0_advisory_
board.php

Campbell's Center for Nutrition and Wellness (Campbell's Soup)

Gatorade Sports Science Institute (PepsiCo owns Gatorade)
www.gssiweb.com

Global Advisory Council on Balanced Lifestyles (McDonald's)
www.mcdonalds.com/corp/values/socialrespons/resrecog/expert_
advisors0/advisory_council_on.html

Hershey Center for Health and Nutrition (yes, as in the chocolate company)

International Life Sciences Institute
Funded by member corporations; works to undermine global nutrition
policy.
www.ilsi.org

Worldwide Health & Wellness Advisory Council (Kraft Foods)
www.kraft.com/obesity/advisory.html

Corporate Educational Wellness Programs

Balance First
PepsiCo's program aimed at elementary schools.
www.smartspot.com/balancefirst/4-3_balance_first.php

Balanced for Life
National Automatic Merchandising Association's Web site.
www.balancedforlife.net

Brand New You
General Mills' weight-loss program.
www.brandnewyou.com

Get Active Stay Active
Web-based program sponsored by PepsiCo; recipient of the President's
Challenge Physical Activity and Fitness Awards Program.
www.getactivestayactive.com

Girls on the Run
Sponsored by Kellogg's Frosted Flakes and New Balance athletic footwear
company.
www.girlsontherun.org

Get Fit Challenge
Kellogg's twelve-week program. Step one: "Eat one serving of Kellogg's
cereal per day."
www.kelloggs.com/promotions/getinstep/index.shtml

Kidnetic.com
Funded by numerous corporations and industry groups, including the International Food Information Council and the International Life Sciences Institute.

Live-It!, Step With It, and *Fit It In*
Coca-Cola's in-school programs.
www.liveitprogram.com

Passport to Play
McDonald's in-school program.
www.mcdonalds.com/usa/good/balanced__active_lifestyles.html

S.M.A.R.T. Living
PepsiCo's Web-based program connected to its "Smart Spot."
www.smartspot.com/2_smart_living/2-0_home.php

Salsa, Sabor y Salud
Kraft Foods' "healthy lifestyles program for Latino families."
www.nlci.org/salsa/indexSSS.htm

Weekly Reader MyPyramid
Grocery Manufacturers Association's curriculum on the food guide
pyramid.
www.gmabrands.com/news/docs/NewsRelease.cfm?DocID=1569

Public–Private Partnerships

America on the Move
The Web site's claim that "[i]t's all about energy balance" tells all; the
two main corporate sponsors are PepsiCo and (meat packer) Cargill.
www.americaonthemove.org

Champions for Healthy Kids
Grant program established by General Mills in partnership with the
American Dietetic Association Foundation and the President's Challenge.
www.generalmills.com/corporate/commitment/champions.aspx

Coalition for a Healthy and Active America
Founders include a Cola-Cola executive; note key phrases under
"founding principles": "Commitment to Fitness" and "Freedom of
Choice."
www.chaausa.org

Coalition for Healthy Children
Spearheaded by the Ad Council to provide consistent "messaging"; sponsors include Coca-Cola, General Mills, Kellogg, Kraft Foods, and PepsiCo.
http://healthychildren.adcouncil.org

Get Kids in Action
Partnership between Gatorade (owned by PepsiCo) and the University of
North Carolina Chapel Hill.
www.getkidsinaction.org

President's Challenge
In collaboration with "General Mills Community Action," free presiden-
tial recognition awards are provided to "eligible low-socioeconomic-status
schools."
www.presidentschallenge.org

Shaping America's Youth
Collects information for national database and conducts public forums on
overweight among children; sponsors include Cadbury Schweppes,
Campbell Soup Company, and McNeil Nutritionals (maker of the artificial sweetener Splenda).
www.shapingamericasyouth.com

Industry Newsletters

The Food Institute Daily Update
www.foodinstitute.com

Smart Brief (sponsored by the National Restaurant
Association)
www.smartbrief.com/nra

MYTH VS. REALITY
Nutrition Labeling at Fast-Food and Other Chain Restaurants

In opposing commonsense laws to require chain restaurants to post basic nutrition information, the restaurant industry has perpetuated a number of myths. Here are the most common examples, and suggestions for how to respond.[1]

Myth: Restaurant nutrition labeling will force mom-and-pop restaurants out of business.
Reality: The proposed legislation would apply only to restaurants that belong to chains with ten or more outlets. Small-business owners would not be affected by this legislation.

Myth: Special orders are common, and it would be impossible for a menu to list nutrition information for all possible different food-preparation options and combinations.
Reality: The bill would require fast-food and other chain restaurants to provide nutrition information for menu items as "offered for sale." It does not apply to customized orders or to daily specials (which are not standard menu items). If restaurants can provide nutrition information on Web sites and brochures, they should be able to do so on menus and menu boards. Even if people customize their orders, providing nutrition information for standard menu items at chain restaurants would provide a good basis for comparison from which customers could make informed choices.

Myth: The current system of voluntary labeling at restaurants is adequate.
Reality: Under the current system of voluntary labeling, half of the largest chain restaurants do not provide any nutrition information about their food to their customers. We know of no restaurants that provide calorie labeling for all menu items directly on menus or menu boards. A system requiring

all chain restaurants to provide nutritional information on menus and menu boards would provide a level playing field in a highly competitive industry.

Myth: People already have access to nutrition labeling at restaurants.
Reality: The approximately one-half of restaurants that do provide nutrition information usually do so on Web sites, which have to be accessed before leaving for the restaurant, or on hard-to-find and difficult-to-read posters or brochures in their stores. Placing the nutrition information on the menu or menu board would be right at the point of decision making, and thus more convenient and easier to use.

Myth: Nutrition labeling at fast-food and other chain restaurants will not help to reduce obesity because people eat out so infrequently.
Reality: Americans are relying increasingly on restaurants to feed themselves and their families—restaurants are not just for special occasions anymore. In fact, Americans are eating out twice as much as in 1970. Adults and children get about one-third of their calories from restaurants and other food-service establishments. On a typical day, the National Restaurant Association (NRA) estimates that more than four out of ten adults patronize restaurants.

Providing nutrition information at chain restaurants would allow people to make informed choices for a significant and growing part of their diets. Eating out is associated with higher calorie intakes and higher body weights. Children eat almost twice as many calories when they eat a meal at a restaurant as compared to eating at home (770 versus 420 calories). Portion sizes at restaurants are often large and, for just a little more money, customers can upgrade to larger serving sizes. Restaurant meals often provide a half to a whole day's worth of calories.

Myth: When people eat out they want to splurge and do not want nutrition information.
Reality: While people may choose to ignore nutrition information on certain occasions, two-thirds of Americans support requiring restaurants to list nutrition information, such as calories, on menus, according to four nationally representative surveys.

Myth: The cost of nutrition labeling would drive chain restaurants out of business.
Reality: Half of the largest chain restaurants already provide nutrition information on their Web sites and would not incur any new costs for analyzing their products. The cost to have a product analyzed is about $230

per menu item. A restaurant chain with eighty menu items would incur a *one-time* cost of approximately $18,000 to have all its menu items tested—which would amount to less than ten dollars for each Denny's outlet. The cost of redesigning menus and menu boards would be modest. Many chain restaurants centralize menu development and printing, and restaurant headquarters incur the costs.

Myth: Nutrition labeling at restaurants is a radical idea advocated by the "food police" trying to tell us what we can and cannot eat.
Reality: Nutrition labeling would not limit choices at restaurants. It simply would provide information regarding those choices. Supporters of better nutrition information at restaurants include:

- The U.S. surgeon general and Department of Health and Human Services' "Call to Action" on obesity recommends "increasing availability of nutrition information for foods eaten and prepared away from home."
- Seventeen cities, states, and territories have introduced legislation to require better nutrition information at fast-food and other chain restaurants.
- Two-thirds of Americans support requiring nutrition labeling of restaurant foods.

Myth: Nutrition labeling on packaged foods in supermarkets has not been effective in helping people to make healthier food choices.
Reality: Americans rank nutrition second only to taste as the factor most frequently influencing food purchases. Three-fourths of adults report using food labels. People who read nutrition labels are more likely to have a diet lower in fat and cholesterol and higher in vitamin C. Also, packaged-food labeling has resulted in reformulation of existing products to improve their nutritional quality, as well as the introduction of new, nutritionally improved (low-fat, low-sodium, etc.) products. Finally, the rise in obesity rates began well before "Nutrition Facts" labels were required on packaged foods. "Nutrition Facts" labels have only been required on packaged foods since 1994. Obesity rates started to increase in 1980.

Myth: Menu labeling is not necessary because restaurants already provide a wide variety of foods to meet any individual's dietary needs.
Reality: The nutritional quality of restaurant meals varies and a range of options is usually available. However, without nutrition information, it is

difficult to compare options and make informed decisions. Studies show that estimating the calorie and fat content of restaurant foods is difficult, even for nutrition professionals. Few people would guess that a tuna salad sandwich from a typical deli has 50 percent more calories than a roast beef with mustard sandwich, or that a small milkshake has more calories than a Big Mac.

Myth: Physical inactivity is primarily responsible for obesity—unhealthy eating habits play only a minor role.

Reality: The high levels of obesity in the United States are attributable to both unhealthy eating and physical inactivity, and both must be addressed to help reduce obesity, heart disease, cancer, and other diseases. Most Americans are not getting the recommended amount of physical activity. However, existing data and societal trends suggest that activity levels were already low by 1980, when obesity rates started to increase. Many major societal trends leading to decreased physical activity occurred before 1980—the move to the suburbs, shift to an information economy and more desk jobs, reliance on the car, and the wide availability of labor-saving devices. It is not clear whether further declines in physical activity have occurred since then.

In contrast, the data and societal trends are clear regarding the importance of increased caloric intake in driving the rising obesity rates. National surveys and food-supply data show that adults and children are consuming more calories (about 168 more calories per day for men and 335 more calories per day for women between 1971 and 2000). In addition, since 1980, there have been increases in portion sizes, eating out, and soft drink intake. It would require a great deal of physical activity to burn off the calories consumed in many popular restaurant foods and meals.

Thanks to the Center for Science in the Public Interest for this analysis.

Appendix 4

TAKING BACK OUR SCHOOLS

Advice from Advocates

Based on my extensive interviews with advocates from around the country who have been involved in the on-the-ground battles to get state bills passed to improve school nutrition, I have gleaned the following:

Find a strong legislative ally who is not willing to compromise

The few victories that have been won were in large part due to dedicated politicians not willing to give up the fight.

Don't try to include too much in your bill

While different states are using different strategies, California found success by going after beverages separately from food. This helped to divide the companies, and thus diminished their lobbying strength.

Take the time to build a strong coalition

Connecticut's Lucy Nolan gathered an incredible array of support. She says to make sure that all the groups that are interested in the passage of the bill are also pushing for it.

Reframe the debate

Maine representative Sean Faircloth is turning the tables on industry's freedom rhetoric. He's calling for "freedom from commercialization of public schools" by having schools offer healthy choices in vending machines.

Use dramatic visuals

Kentucky's Carolyn Dennis uses sugar models. For example, she takes empty bottles of Coke or Pepsi and fills them with the amount of sugar they contain. She's says:

"Even more dramatic is a heavy-duty ziplock bag, filled with 11.5 cups of sugar, which is the equivalent of what you get from drinking one 20-ounce Coke or Pepsi every day for a month, just one a day. This big bag is very impressive; it catches people's attention. I have had legislators tell me, 'I can't get that out of my mind, I keep thinking about that.' "

Get your legislators' attention any way you can

Dennis says that while it's important to stress health, you also have to know your audience. "We have a lot of good old boys in the legislature, older white men. I was talking about diabetes and I said, 'A lot of people don't know that within ten years of onset, 50 percent of males are likely to become impotent.' When I first said it, there was a pause, and I said, 'Let me repeat that.' And Representative Burch stuck his head around a post that was blocking his view and said, 'Carolyn, you got my attention.' And I said, 'Yes, sir, I thought it would!' "

Have a good media strategy and a consistent message

The media likes the "David vs. Goliath" angle, so emphasize the parents vs. soda companies and the parents vs. the schools battle. Also use a consistent message. In Connecticut, the message was: "Protect children, not profits."

Expose the lobbying

Once the corporate lobbying gets out into the public eye, its impact won't be as strong. You can expose the money spent on lobbying state by state by Coca-Cola, PepsiCo, and the Grocery Manufacturers Association, by campaign contributions to lawmakers and by payments to lobbyists—that is, how much money is spent to oppose a certain bill. Also, look at where the companies are strategically putting their money, especially with the political leadership. For example, in Connecticut, it was probably no coincidence that Coke donated a scoreboard in the town where the speaker of the house lives.

Battling industry is a full-time job

Kentucky's Carolyn Dennis says you need to have someone in the capitol on a daily basis. "Because to understand what's going on, you need to know the players, you need to know who the lobbyists are, and who you're up against. You need to be constantly talking to legislators. Corporate lobbyists have such an advantage because they are there every day and all year long and they develop relationships with legislators."

Always be respectful and develop relationships

Dennis says that no matter how you feel about legislators or how much you disagree, always be polite. "If you disagree, say, 'I need to go and think about that' and come back and talk to them later, because it can be hard to think on your feet. They would be surprised because I would come back. It's all about forming relationships with people—the more allies you can build, and the more respectful you are with people. I keep my little book with all the photos of the legislators so I can tell one old white guy from the next. And I stalk them in the halls."

Realize it's a long haul

California's Amanda Purcell says it takes a long time to build consensus around this issue. In California, groups had been working on school nutrition for seven to ten years, getting local policies passed, proving it can work. She says that other states are where California was five years ago. "All the schools were opposed; it was mayhem. It takes coming back, adding another supporter, adding another local example, really building a coalition of organizations." All this takes time.

How Parents Can Get Involved

Advocates need parents and teachers to help ensure that nutrition policies get passed and then implemented. Don't underestimate the power that parents have at both the local school district level and at the state level to demand changes in the nutrition environment of your children's schools.

TRY THIS FOUR-STEP PROCESS:
1. Find out what's happening in your school. What food and beverages are currently being offered to students? What vending contracts are currently in place or being considered? Ask to see them. Try to conduct a survey or walk-through. Look out for marketing schemes such as raffles or giveaways.
2. Form a committee, even if it's just a few parents. Build a broader coalition by bringing in health professionals and others. The federal government now requires that all schools participating in the National School Lunch Program have in place a "wellness policy" that includes nutrition. Use this law to motivate action.
3. Meet with the school district and your elected officials. At the state level, parents can call and write legislators to demand that their schools change.

4. When you're ready, contact the media. For example, go to school board meetings armed with a bag full of junk food products that your kids bought at school, or bags of sugar that represent the amount in sodas.

How to Counter Common Arguments for Soda in Schools

Here is a list of counterarguments that you can adapt to your school situation.

They say: Schools need the money from soda sales

Responses:
• Schools should not be making a profit at the expense of children's health.
• Children were not meant to fund their education with their own pocket change.
• Coke and Pepsi make far more money than the schools do on exclusive pouring rights agreements, especially if you consider the amount per student.
• Often, schools lose more money from the school lunch program than what they can make up in soda sales. (For example, in Texas, school districts made $54 million per year, but lost $61 million in reimbursement under the school lunch program. So the soda sales are undermining meal purchases.)
• If Coke and Pepsi really cared about education, they would donate money outright and not require kids to sacrifice their health.
• It makes more sense for schools to have fund-raisers where kids and parents give money to schools directly, instead of giving a portion to Coke and Pepsi.
• Soda companies are not "donating" money to schools at all; rather, they are exploiting schools' need for funds to benefit their own bottom line and build brand loyalty among an impressionable and captive audience.
• The economic incentive for schools to sell more unhealthy sodas is counterproductive to good education and protecting children from harm.
• Many schools are making as much or even more money selling healthier options, such as 100 percent juice and water. (Examples include California, Maine, Minnesota, and Pennsylvania.)
• Schools should not be so cash-strapped as to rely on blood money.
• Schools need to look for better sources of funding for programs.
• Adequate funding of public schools is the responsibility of the government; that is what our taxes are for.

They say: It's all about choices / Children need to learn how to choose

Responses:
- We don't allow cigarette sales in schools so that children can have "choices."
- We restrict children's choices in all sorts of ways in order to protect them.
- Children have plenty of choices once they leave the school grounds.
- Parents are still free to send children to school with sodas for lunch.
- We do have a freedom of choice problem—you can't find a healthy drink! (Paraphrasing Sean Faircloth, Maine state representative.)
- We need to create the best environment for children to make healthy choices.
- If parents want to give their kids a treat, they can do so at home.
- Schools have a responsibility to provide children with healthy choices.
- Kids will make healthy choices if you make those choices available and educate kids about them.
- Exclusive pouring rights agreements actually take away choice. Once the contract is signed, students' choices are limited to that vendor's products.

They say: This is a complex problem / There is no scientific basis

Responses:
- Soda is a significant enough contributor to obesity/diabetes/other health problems that it should be eliminated.
- Saying that any one thing won't solve the problem is no excuse for doing nothing.
- The studies that industry cites as showing no connection between drinking excessive amounts of soda and health problems were funded by industry.
- Soda often displaces nutrients that children need.

They say: Schools should have local control

Responses:
- Schools should have local control when it benefits children, not when it serves to accelerate the sales of Coke and Pepsi. (Paraphrasing the California PTA.)
- We don't allow schools to have local control over things of utmost importance, such as education standards or children's health.
- Children's health is more important than local control.
- In California, the school board association (which usually defends local control) supported a ban on soda in all public schools in that state because of the overriding interest of children's health.

They say: Exercise is the real solution

Responses:
• It's not only about exercising; it's also about eating right.
• One 20-ounce soda has 17 teaspoons of sugar, for a whopping 250 empty calories. A kid who drinks one soda a day for a week would need to bicycle for 4 hours and 20 minutes just to burn off the calories from the soda. (From the California Center for Public Health Advocacy.)
• Ironically, drinking too much soda can actually lead to broken bones; therefore, drinking too much soda can put kids at risk for more activity-related injuries.

They say: Parents are really the problem

Responses:
• Schools act in place of parents for the entire day, five days a week.
• Parents trust schools not to undermine their own education efforts at home.
• Parents should not have to worry about how their children are spending their lunch money.

They say: Students will go outside to buy sodas anyway

Responses:
• Most school campuses are closed; 94 percent of elementary, 89 percent of middle/junior high and 73 percent of high schools have a closed-campus policy. (Source: Center for Science in the Public Interest.)
• Schools should remain a safe haven and educate at every opportunity.

Miscellaneous Arguments: The Importance of Teaching Values
• Schools should be a safe haven from corporate marketing.
• Children are captive at school; they should not be branding opportunities.
• Schools should teach the same values outside and inside the classroom.
• Schools should practice what they preach by supporting and reinforcing nutrition education in the classroom.
• Children learn both by what we tell them and by what we sell them.

Appendix 5

PROTECT YOUR LEGAL RIGHTS

Because the food industry feels threatened by potential lawsuits, trade groups are going state by state to take away your access to the courtroom. Knowing how to respond to their arguments can help oppose this power grab.

Counterarguments to the National Restaurant Association's Talking Points

Argument: Frivolous lawsuits blaming the restaurant industry for obesity in America deny the role that personal responsibility plays in the dietary choices that individuals make on a daily basis.
Response: Keeping litigation available doesn't deny the role of individual dietary choice; it merely represents one potential tool to address the problem.

Argument: Healthy eating should be promoted by knowledge, not lawsuits.
Response: Then the restaurant industry should provide nutrition labeling. Why are the large chains opposing laws and withholding such information?

Argument: With restaurant profit margins averaging around 4 percent, a single frivolous lawsuit is enough to put a small restaurant out of business.
Response: There is no way to substantiate this claim. Anyway, small restaurants are an unlikely target of a lawsuit. This is just another "little guy" scare tactic.

Argument: We need to protect our industry from abusive, frivolous lawsuits and prevent the food industry from being held responsible for the complex issue of obesity. All foods can be part of a healthy lifestyle."
Response: The "complexity" of obesity is another familiar refrain from the food industry. Each solution or strategy is attacked as too simplistic or dismissed because obesity is so complex. The complexity of the issue shouldn't be an excuse to not act at all, but rather is the very reason that we need to

maintain the availability of a wide array of policy solutions. And it's certainly no reason to preclude the rights of consumers to have access to the court system.

Argument: "It is unfortunate, but necessary, to have legislation enacted that will help deter unscrupulous attorneys from filing abusive, frivolous lawsuits that only enrich the trial bar at the expense of the hardworking restaurant operators and their employees."

Response: Here the rhetoric of the evil, greedy trial lawyers is contrasted with the mom-and-pop imagery of the restaurants. No argument is actually made; rather, the rhetoric is intended to suffice.

Additional Counter-Rhetoric—Legal Arguments

Food-industry defense lawyers have created legal arguments in an effort to legitimate the food industry's anticonsumer and anti–public health shield law legislation, while deliberately ignoring critical legal issues. The following will help you highlight some of the flaws in the industry's model legislation.

What They Say

Shield laws are necessary to avoid frivolous lawsuits that make a mockery of the legal and judicial system and overemphasize our culture's victim mentality.

What They Don't Say

State shield laws may be unconstitutional. Most state constitutions provide citizens with access to state courts to redress their grievances and recover compensation for injuries. Food-industry shield laws prevent lawsuits from even being brought; the industry has decided before any arguments can be raised that citizens may not be heard on these issues. In several states, including Florida and Utah, counsel for the state legislature has warned that shield laws may run afoul of state constitutional provisions that guarantee citizens access to the courts. Once passed, unconstitutional laws can remain on the books if they are not challenged in a lawsuit. In Arizona, because a shield law *would* violate the state constitution, legislators had to construct a special defense that could be raised by a food-industry defendant only *after* a citizen exercised his or her constitutional rights to go to court. The present spate of "anti-obesity" shield laws is not the first time the food industry has managed to force protective but likely unconstitutional laws onto the books. In the 1990s, "food disparagement" or "veggie libel laws" were passed to "protect" perishable foods against slander; that is, a citizen could be subject to criminal prosecution and heavy fines for saying "bad" things about certain foods. This protectionist law in Texas was the basis for an unsuccessful lawsuit against Oprah Winfrey for millions of dollars for her reaction to certain unhealthful beef-industry practices.

What They Say

Frivolous obesity lawsuits could overburden the courts and ultimately cost taxpayers millions of dollars in court-related expenses.

What They Don't Say

Food-industry lawyers are prolific litigators when it suits them. Although the food industry is quick to take away citizens' rights to sue, food-industry lawyers file thousands of lawsuits, some of which are frivolous or seek to silence food-industry critics. For example, McDonald's has sued an Italian restaurant reviewer for likening their fries to cardboard and two activists in England for their statements critical of McDonald's practices. The latter lawsuit resulted in "McLibel," the longest (ten-plus years) trial in British history.

What They Say

Food-industry lawyers argue that obesity-related lawsuits are outside the bounds of traditional tort law that recompenses an injured party for getting sick on spoiled food or for an injury caused by the producers' "failure to warn"—for example, of the presence of peanuts. They also argue that the food industry has been transparent about the content of its products.

What They Don't Say

Obesity lawsuits do fall within traditional tort law parameters. One example is the Pelman lawsuit against McDonald's discussed in Chapter 12. The fast-food industry has a long history of touting its food as healthy and nutritious while encouraging consumers to eat lots of it without any warning that such overconsumption could be harmful. It steadfastly refuses to inform consumers of calorie and nutritional content on menu boards, where the most people are likely to see it. Fast-food products are often likely to contain many ingredients that neither the home cook nor the typical consumer would expect. These allegations fit squarely into "traditional" food tort claims. While food-related tort law traditionally affects a limited number of people, even in a major outbreak, the number of people, including children and adults, suffering from obesity is huge. Class action lawsuits were intended to both recompense a public that has been injured *and* create change when legislators refused to act in the public interest. They, too, have become a "traditional" tort law tool.

Thanks to the Public Health Advocacy Institute, which collaborated on this project.

RESOURCES FOR POSITIVE CHANGE

There are hundreds of groups around the country doing inspiring work to improve the food system. Here are a few of my favorite groups, which you can support and call upon for more resources.

National Organizations—Nutrition and Children's Advocacy

Campaign for a Commercial-Free Childhood

A coalition of groups, professionals, and parents working to counter the harmful effects of all forms of marketing to children, including junk food.
www.commercialexploitation.org

Center for Informed Food Choices

My own organization, which promotes a whole-foods, plant-based diet and educates about the politics of food; sign up for the blog update.
www.informedeating.org

Center for Science in the Public Interest

For decades, CSPI has been pushing for stronger nutrition policies.
www.cspinet.org

CHOICE: Citizens for Healthy Options in Children's Education

Provides numerous resources to promote plant-based meals in schools.
www.choiceusa.net

Commercial Alert

Works to minimize the impact of commercialism, especially on children's health.
www.commercialalert.org

Community Food Security Coalition

A coalition of groups that address the lack of fresh, affordable, and sustainable healthy food in low-income communities by improving food systems.
www.foodsecurity.org

The Food Studies Institute

Improving children's diets through an innovative and award-winning curriculum that engages kids in sensory-based, hands-on learning.
www.foodstudies.org

GRACE Factory Farm Project

Works to create a sustainable food system that is healthful and humane.
www.factoryfarm.org

Health Care Without Harm

Working with hospitals to provide nutritious food from sustainable sources.
www.noharm.org

Institute for Agriculture and Trade Policy

Promotes family farms and sustainable agriculture through research and advocacy; authors of the excellent 2006 report, "Food without Thought: How U.S. Farm Policy Contributes to Obesity."
www.iatp.org
www.agobservatory.org

National Farm to School Program

A project of the Center for Food and Justice at Occidental College (California); more than four hundred farm-to-school programs in twenty-two states connect local farms with school cafeterias; a similar program is called farm-to-college.
www.farmtoschool.org
www.farmtocollege.org

Parents Against Junk Food

Started by the editor of PBS's *America's Test Kitchen*, this nonprofit is devoted to the elimination of junk food from public schools.
www.parentsagainstjunkfood.org

Physicians Committee for Responsible Medicine

Promotes preventive medicine through vegetarian diets; also works to reform federal nutrition policy and uses legal tools to protect consumers.
www.pcrm.org

Public Health Advocacy Institute

Working to advance public health through legal and policy tools; "Law and Obesity" project offers resources for preserving consumers' access to the courts.
www.phaionline.org

Organic Consumers Association

Works to protect the integrity of organic standards, preserve the environment, and promote locally grown, sustainable food.
www.organicconsumers.org

Small Planet Institute

Founded by authors Frances Moore Lappé (*Diet for a Small Planet*, *Democracy's Edge*, among many other books) and Anna Lappé (*Hope's Edge*, *Grub*) to promote "living democracy" and share inspirational stories from around the world.
www.smallplanetinstitute.org

State and Local Groups

California Center for Public Health Advocacy

Led the effort to pass legislation to improve school food in California.
www.publichealthadvocacy.org

California Food and Justice Coalition

Working to create a healthy and just food system.
www.foodsecurity.org/california

California Project LEAN

Numerous resources, including "Taking the Fizz out of Soda Contracts: A Guide to Community Action" and "An Action Guide to Stop the Marketing of Unhealthy Food and Beverages in Schools."
www.californiaprojectlean.org

Coalition of Immokalee Workers

Based in southern Florida, this dedicated group of immigrant farm workers is organizing successful campaigns against fast-food giants such as Taco Bell and McDonald's for improved living conditions.
www.ciw-online.org

Food Policy Blog

Maintained by Parke Wilde, a food economist at Tufts University, who expertly reveals the politics behind the policymaking.
www.usfoodpolicy.blogspot.com

The Food Project

Youth-focused programs that focus on sustainable agriculture in Massachusetts.
www.thefoodproject.org

The Food Trust

Numerous inspiring campaigns in both schools and communities to, for example, increase access to supermarkets in low-income neighborhoods in Pennsylvania.
www.thefoodtrust.org

Just Food

Working to develop a just and sustainable food system in New York City.
www.justfood.org

Massachusetts Public Health Association

Published an excellent organizing tool: "Community Action to Change School Food Policy."
www.mphaweb.org

No Junk Food

Providing resources to inspire others to follow the lead of the Los Angeles Unified School District, which was the first to ban soda and junk food.
www.nojunkfood.org

Oregon Public Health Institute

Published an excellent review of soda contracts in Oregon public schools.
www.communityhealthpartnership.org

The People's Grocery

Numerous innovative, community-based and youth-focused programs to bring fresh health food to West Oakland, California.
www.peoplesgrocery.org

International Groups

Agribusiness Accountability Initiative

An international network of experts that recognize how corporations threaten the sustainability of the global food system; provides a clearing-house of resources.
www.agribusinessaccountability.org

Feed Me Better Campaign

The "Naked Chef" Jamie Oliver's one-man crusade to improve school meals in England and beyond; provides resources for change.
www.feedmebetter.com

Food Commission

An independent organization campaigning for safer and healthier food in the UK.
www.foodcomm.org.uk

Food First

The Institute for Food Development and Policy works to eliminate the injustices that cause hunger by reshaping the global food system.
www.foodfirst.org

Food Secure Canada

Works to provide healthy, sustainable food to everyone in a dignified manner.
www.foodsecurecanada.org

GM Watch

Devoted to exposing the propaganda, PR, front groups, and lobbyists used by industry to promote genetic modification; especially concerned with Africa.
www.gmwatch.org

India Resource Center

Supports movements against globalization in India; particularly active in opposing the environmental destruction caused by Coca-Cola.
www.indiaresource.org

International Food Policy Research Institute

Working to achieve sustainable food security and reduce poverty in developing countries; publishes numerous reports and resources.
www.ifpri.org

Sustain: The Alliance for Better Food and Farming

A UK-based coalition that advocates food and agriculture policies and practices that enhance the health and welfare of people and animals.
www.sustainweb.org

Tracking Legislation and Lobbying

Center for Media and Democracy

Publishers of *PR Watch*, the *Weekly Spin*, and *SourceWatch*, invaluable tools for keeping up with the public relations industry, getting behind the spin, and understanding how corporations and government shape public opinion.
www.prwatch.org
www.sourcewatch.org

Center for Public Integrity

Provides resources on state lobbying through its "Hired Guns" project.
www.publicintegrity.org

Center for Responsive Politics

Searchable databases of federal and state campaign donations organized by official, industry, and corporation.
www.opensecrets.org

ConsumerDeception.com

An excellent Web site created by People for the Ethical Treatment of Animals that exposes the truth behind the industry front group Center for Consumer Freedom.
www.consumerdeception.com

Corporate Accountability Project

Numerous resources on researching corporations and campaign donations.
www.corporations.org

Freedom of Information Center

Resources include sample letters on filing "freedom of information act"
(FOIA) requests—for example, to obtain copies of school soda contracts.
http://foi.missouri.edu/foialett.html
See also: *FOIA Advocates*
www.foiadvocates.com

The Institute on Money in State Politics

Probably the most comprehensive database on state lobbying money.
www.followthemoney.org

National Conference of State Legislatures

A bipartisan organization that tracks state bills and writes reports.
www.ncsl.org

National Restaurant Association

Industry trade group, reliable for tracking the bills they lobby for and
against.
www.restaurant.org

Program on Corporations, Law and Democracy

Provides wonderful resources on how corporations operate.
www.poclad.org

ReclaimDemocracy.org

Dedicated to restoring democratic authority over corporations and reviving
grassroots democracy.
www.reclaimdemocracy.org

ENDNOTES

INTRODUCTION

1. See e.g., David Suzuki, "Thrifty Gene Can Be Costly," *Science Matters*, June 13, 2003.
2. USDA Factbook, Chapter 2, "Profiling Food Consumption in America." www.usda.gov/factbook/chapter2.pdf.
3. Joel Furhman, *Disease-Proof Your Child: Feeding Kids Right* (New York: St. Martin's Press, 2005), 10.
4. S. Boyd Eaton and Stanley Eaton, "Evolution, Diet and Health," paper presented at the 14th International Congress of Anthropological and Ethnological Sciences. www.cast.uark.edu/local/icaes/conferences/wburg/posters/sboydeaton/eaton.htm.
5. See e.g., U.S. Department of Agriculture, "America's Eating Habits, Changes and Consequences: An Economic Research Service Report," April 1999. http://www.ers.usda.gov/Publications/aib750/.
6. Joanne F. Guthrie, "Understanding Fruit and Vegetable Choices: Economic and Behavioral Influences," *Agriculture Information Bulletin* AIB792-1, November 2004.
7. Center for Science in the Public Interest, "Liquid Candy: How Soft Drinks are Harming America's Health," 2005. http://www.cspinet.org/liquidcandy/.
8. Eaton and Eaton, "Evolution, Diet and Health."
9. USDA Factbook, Chapter 2, "Profiling Food Consumption in America."
10. Ibid.
11. U.S. Department of Health and Human Services, "The Surgeon General's Call to Action to Prevent and Decrease Overweight and Obesity," 2001. http://www.surgeongeneral.gov/topics/obesity/calltoaction/CalltoAction.pdf.
12. Associated Press, "Study: Number of Overweight Kids to Increase Sharply," *USA Today*, March 5, 2006.
13. Worldwatch Institute, news release, "Chronic Hunger and Obesity Epidemic Eroding Global Progress," March 2004. www.worldwatch.org/press/news/2000/03/04/.
14. Cardiovascular diseases include high blood pressure, coronary heart disease, congestive heart failure, and stroke, among others. See American Heart Association News, "Cardiovascular Statistics Updated for 2005: New Data

on Risk Factors in America's Youth," December 30, 2004. www.american-heart.org/presenter.jhtml?identifier=3027696.

15. U.S. Department of Health and Human Services, "The Surgeon General's Call to Action to Prevent and Decrease Overweight and Obesity," 10.

16. Marion Nestle, quoted in: J.M. Hirsch, "Food Industry a Target in Obesity Fight," March 19, 2006. www.forbes.com/feeds/ap/2006/03/18/ap260 5096.html.

17. Grocery Manufacturers Association Web site: www.gmabrands.com.

18. National Restaurant Association Web site: www.restaurant.org/aboutus/.

CHAPTER 1

1. See e.g., Kelly D. Brownell and Katherine Battle Horgen, *Food Fight* (New York: McGraw-Hill, 2003).

2. Frank H. Easterbrook and Daniel R. Fishel, "Antitrust Suits by Targets of Tender Offers," *Michigan Law Review* (1982): 1177, quoted in Joel Bakan, *The Corporation* (New York: Free Press, 2004).

3. Chris Laszlo, *The Sustainable Company* (Washington, D.C.: Island Press, 2003), 46.

4. Lee Allen, telephone conversion with author, February 15, 2006.

5. Ibid.

6. Jerry Mander, "The Rules of Corporate Behavior," in *The Case Against the Global Economy* (San Francisco: Sierra Club Books, 1996), 320.

7. Erik Assadourian, "The Role of Stakeholders in the Evolving Corporation," online discussion at: www.worldwatch.org/live/discussion/113/.

8. Lee Allen conversation.

9. Ibid.

10. Ibid.

11. Joel Bakan, *The Corporation*, 109-10.

12. American Beverage Association, press release, "Beverage Industry Announces New School Vending Policy," August 16, 2005. www.ameribev.org/press-room/2005_vending.asp.

13. Editorial, "Soft Drink Industry Takes High Road," *Atlanta Journal-Constitution*, August 18, 2005. (The *Atlanta Journal-Constitution* is the hometown paper of Coca-Cola.)

14. Associated Press with Tom Paulson and Gregory Roberts, "Schools Get Ally in Soda Issue: Drink Makers," *Seattle Post-Intelligencer*, August 17, 2005.

15. Child Health News "U.S. Beverage Industry Praised for Helping in Childhood Obesity," News-Medical.net, August 17, 2005. www.news-medical.net/?id=12549.

16. ABA press release.

17. Elliot Maras, "Beverage Industry Group Supports Limiting Carbonated Soda in Schools," *Vending Market Watch*, August 17, 2005.

18. Editorial, "Soft Drink Industry Takes High Road," *Atlanta Journal-Constitution*, August 18, 2005.

19. Todd Dorman, "Vilsack: Educate Kids on Making Good Food Choices," *Quad-City Times*, February 16, 2006.

20. Tracy Jan, "A Sweet Tooth Is Tough to Pull: Even When Schools Ban Candy Machines, Pupils Indulge," *Boston Globe*, February 15, 2006.
21. ABA press release.
22. Clinton Foundation press release, May 3, 2006. www.clintonfoundation.org/ 050306-nr-cf-hs-hk-usa-pr-healthy-school-beverage-guidelines-set-for-united-states-schools.htm.
23. These states at press time include Massachusetts and Rhode Island.

CHAPTER 2

1. Shelly Rosen, remarks at the *Time*/ABC Summit on Obesity, June 3, 2004. A Web cast is available at www.rwjf.org.
2. Ric Keller Web site, news item, "Keller's Food Liability Reform Bill Passes House with Bipartisan Support," October 18, 2005. http://keller. house.gov/News/DocumentSingle.aspx?DocumentID=35677.
3. National Restaurant Association, news release, "National Restaurant Association Announces Strong Support for 'Personal Responsibility in Food Consumption Act,'" April 29, 2005. www.restaurant.org/pressroom/pressrelease. cfm?ID=1079.
4. Center for Consumer Freedom "About Us" Web page: www.consumerfreedom. com/about.cfm.
5. Michele Simon biography on ActivistCash: www.activistcash.com/biography.cfm/bid/3539.
6. CCF advertisement. www.consumerfreedom.com/advertisements_detail.cfm/ad/7.
7. GMA, news release, "GMA Statement Regarding IOM Report on Food Marketing to Children," December 6, 2005. www.gmabrands.com/news/docs/ NewsRelease.cfm?DocID=1588.
8. See e.g., Jean Kilbourne, *Can't Buy My Love* (New York: Touchstone Books, 1999).
9. ABA, press release, "NSDA Statement on Efforts to Ban or Restrict the Sale of Carbonated Soft Drinks in Schools," August 27, 2002. http://ameribev.org/ pressroom/2002_statementonbans.asp.
10. GMA, news release, March 16, 2005. www.gmabrands.com/news/docs/ NewsRelease.cfm?DocID=1466.
11. Dan Mindus, letter to the editor, "Harvard Study on Fitness Misleading," *Boston Globe*, December 31, 2004.
12. Shelly Rosen, remarks at the *Time*/ABC Summit on Obesity.
13. ACFN, Testimony before House Government Reform Committee, Washington, D.C., June 3, 2004. http://www.acfn.org/pressrelease/060304/.
14. GMA, "GMA Testimony in Opposition to Maryland School Marketing Bill," March 12, 2003. www.gmabrands.com/news/docs/Testimony.cfm?docid= 1091.
15. PepsiCo Web site: www.smartspot.ca/energy_balance.php.
16. Linda Bacon, e-mail message to author, March 9, 2006.
17. Caroline E. Mayer, "Work Off Those Cheetos!" *Washington Post*, November 23, 2005.

18. Ibid.
19. Pepsico, news release, "PepsiCo Reports Strong Sales and Operating Results for 2005 Fourth Quarter and Full Year," February 8, 2005. http://phx.corporate-ir.net/phoenix.zhtml?c=78265&p=irol-newsArticle_Print&ID=814075&highlight.
20. Caroline E. Mayer, "Work Off Those Cheetos!"
21. Caroline E. Mayer, "McDonald's Makes Ronald a Health Ambassador," *Washington Post*, January 28, 2005.
22. Reuters, "Ronald McDonald Gets an Extreme Makeover," June 9, 2005. http://msnbc.msn.com/id/8135239.
23. Associated Press, "McDonald's Gives Ronald Jock Makeover to Fit with Healthier Menu," June 9, 2005.
24. Associated Press, "Ronald McJock? McDonald's Gives Mascot a Sporty Look," June 10, 2005.
25. Reuters, "Ronald McDonald Gets an Extreme Makeover."
26. McDonald's, news release, "McDonald's Teams Up with Educators and Health/Nutrition Experts to Promote Balanced, Active Lifestyles in Schools," August 23, 2005. www.primezone.com/newsroom/news.html?d=84367.
27. McDonald's, news release, "McDonald's Passport to Play Kicks Off in 31,000 U.S. Schools," September 13, 2005. http://www.hispanicprwire.com/news.php?l=in&id=4789&cha=9.
28. Susan Linn, e-mail message to author, March 20, 2005.
29. Coca-Cola, news release. www2.coca-cola.com/presscenter/nr_20050526_americas_liveit.html.
30. Coca-Cola, Live It! Fact Sheet. www.yourpowertochoose.com/word/Live_It!_Fact_Sheet.pdf.
31. SourceWatch.org entry on Coca-Cola. www.sourcewatch.org/index.php?title=Coca-Cola.
32. Joe Hughes, "Firefighter Chosen for Live-Healthy Campaign," *San Diego Union-Tribune*, February 14, 2005.
33. "GMA Testimony in Opposition to Maryland School Marketing Bill."
34. Richard Daynard, telephone conversation with author, February 19, 2006.

CHAPTER 3

1. Richard Berman interview in *Chain Leader*, as quoted in Sheldon Rampton and John Stauber, "Berman & Co.: 'Nonprofit' Hustlers for the Food & Booze Biz," *PR Watch*, Vol. 8, No. 1. www.prwatch.org/prwissues/2001Q1/berman1.html.
2. Sheldon Rampton and John Stauber, "ConsumerFreedom.org: Tobacco Money Takes on Activist Cash," *PR Watch*, Vol. 9, No. 1. www.prwatch.org/prwissues/2002Q1/ddam.html.
3. Documents compiled on the PETA Web site, ConsumerDeception.com: www.consumerdeception.com/append4.html.
4. Caroline E. Mayer and Amy Joyce, "The Escalating Obesity Wars," *Washington*

Post, April 27, 2005. www.citizensforethics.org/press/pressclip. php?view=167.

5. PCRM, news release, "Physicians' Group Responds to Smear Tactics by Tobacco/Meat Industry Front Group," November 7, 2005. www.pcrm. org/news/pcrmresponds.html.

6. Center for Consumer Freedom Web site: www.consumerfreedom.com/about.cfm.

7. Center for Consumer Freedom Web site: www.consumerfreedom.com/advertisements_detail.cfm/ad/38.

8. List compiled on the PETA Web site, ConsumerDeception.com: www.consumerdeception.com/append3.html.

9. Center for Consumer Freedom Web site, CSPIScam.com: www.cspiscam.com/.

10. Center for Consumer Freedom Web site; www.consumerfreedom.com/about.cfm.

11. Marion Nestle biography on Center for Consumer Freedom Web site: www.activistcash.com/biography.cfm/bid/3381.

12. Marion Nestle, e-mail message to author, March 16, 2006.

13. Michele Simon biography on Center for Consumer Freedom Web site: www.activistcash.com/biography.cfm/bid/3539.

14. SourceWatch.org entry on Center for Consumer Freedom: www.sourcewatch.org/wiki.phtml?title=Center_for_Consumer_Freedom#Contributions.

15. CREW, Executive Summary of "CREW Files IRS Complaint against the Center for Consumer Freedom Alleging Violations of Tax-Exempt Status," November 16, 2004. www.citizensforethics.org/activities/campaign.php?view=3.

16. CREW, press release, "CREW Files IRS Complaint Against the Center for Consumer Freedom Alleging Violations of Tax-Exempt Status," November 16, 2004. www.citizensforethics.org/press/newsrelease.php?view=5.

17. SourceWatch.org entry on Center for Consumer Freedom.

18. Center for Consumer Freedom Web site: www.consumerfreedom.com/about.cfm.

19. Bob Burton, e-mail message to author, March 14, 2006.

20. Richard Daynard, telephone conversation with author, February 19, 2006.

21. SourceWatch.org entry on Center for Consumer Freedom.

CHAPTER 4

1. "Big Mac's Makeover," *The Economist*, October 14, 2004.

2. Associated Press, "McSupersizes to Be Phased Out," March 3, 2004. www.cnn.com/2004/US/03/02/mcdonalds.supersize.ap/.

3. Karen Robinson-Jacobs, "McDonald's Plans to Drop Super Size Fries, Sodas," *Dallas Morning News*, March 17, 2004.

4. Eric Herman, "McDonald's Giant Drinks Return," *Chicago Sun-Times*, June 17, 2005.

5. Andrew Buncombe, "McDonald's Faces Payout over Beef Fat on Its Fries," *The Independent*, March 8, 2002.

6. Associated Press, "McDonald's Facing Lawsuits over French Fries," February 20, 2006. http://www.msnbc.msn.com/id/11459132/from/RSS/.

7. Stephen Joseph, conversation with author, February 7, 2006.

8. $1.5 million was to be used to notify consumers that the oil still contained trans fat, with the remainder donated to the American Heart Association. "Plaintiffs' Press Release on Settlement of McDonald's Trans Fat Litigation" (February 11, 2005). http://www.bantransfats.com/mcdonalds.html.

9. Jeremy Grant, "McDonald's Reveals Higher of Trans Fats Level in Fries," *Financial Times*, February 8, 2006.

10. McDonald's, press release, April 15, 2004. www.mcdonalds.com/usa/news/2004/conpr_04152004.html.

11. The halo effect is defined by Merriam-Webster Online as: "Generalization from the perception of one outstanding personality trait to an overly favorable evaluation of the whole personality." http://m-w.com/cgi-bin/dictionary?book=Dictionary&va=halo%20effect.

12. McDonald's Web site: www.mcdonalds.com/corp/values/balance.html.

13. PCRM report, "The New 'Salads': The Latest in Fast Fraud," May 2003, at: www.pcrm.org/news/health030508.pdf.

14. Brie Turner-McGrievy, e-mail to author, March 29, 2006.

15. Margaret Webb Pressler, "Hold the Health, Serve that Burger," *Washington Post*, August 18, 2005.

16. McDonald's Web site: www.mcdonalds.com/usa/eat/features/salads.html.

17. Pallavi Gogoi, "McDonald's New Wrap," *BusinessWeek Online*, February 17, 2006. http://www.businessweek.com/bwdaily/dnflash/feb2006/nf20060217_8392_db016.htm.

18. McDonald's Web site: www.mcdonalds.com/app_controller.nutrition.index1.html.

19. McDonald's, press release, "McDonald's Debuts 'What's New for Spring' and Announces One of the Hottest Tickets for This Summer," May 9, 2005. http://www.mcdonalds.com/usa/news/2005/conpr_05042005.html.

20. McDonald's, press release, "Launch of McDonald's Fruit and Walnut Salad," May 9, 2005. www.venuswilliams.com/news/fullstory.sps?iNewsid=174250&itype=&iCategoryID=0.

21. McDonald's, press release, "McDonald's Partners with Nutritionist, Author and Motivational Speaker Dr. Ro to Promote 'It's What I Eat and What I Do . . . I'm lovin' It' Public Awareness Campaign," May 4, 2005. www.mcdonalds.com/usa/news/2005/conpr_05092005.html.

22. Campaign for a Commercial-Free Childhood, press release, "Children's Coalition Raps McDonald's Supersized Hypocrisy Hip-Hop Songs to Feature Big Macs," March 24, 2005. www.commondreams.org/news2005/0324-11.htm.

23. David Kiley, "McDonald's Turning Brand Placement into Junk," *BusinessWeek Online*, March 29, 2005, at: www.businessweek.com/the_thread/brand-newday/archives/2005/03/mcdonalds_turni.html.

24. Sabrina Ford, "In a Green Mood," *Alternet*, March 16, 2005. www.alternet.org/wiretap/21507/.

25. Pressler, *Washington Post.*
26. Ibid.
27. Tom Van Riper, "It's the Burgers, Stupid," *Forbes.com*, January 19, 2006. www.forbes.com/business/2006/01/18/mcdonalds-burgers-salads-cx_tvr_0119mcd.html.
28. Pressler, *Washington Post.*
29. "Big Mac's Makeover," *The Economist.*
30. Van Riper, *Forbes.com.*
31. Ibid.
32. "Big Mac's Makeover," *The Economist.*
33. "AC Nielsen Finds U.S. Truly Is a Fast Food Nation," December 21, 2004. http://us.acnielsen.com/news/20041221.shtml.
34. Penelope Patsuris, "McDonald's Is Lovin' Its Turnaround," *Forbes*, December 9, 2004. www.forbes.com/home/commerce/2004/12/09/cx_pp_1209 overachiever.html.
35. Maria Newman, "Walk Off Those Calories: Another Alternative to the Big Mac," *New York Times*, April 15, 2004.
36. National Alliance for Nutrition and Activity, report, "From Wallet to Waistline: The Hidden Costs of 'Super Sizing.'" http://www.preventioninstitute.org/print/portionsizerept.html.
37. A phone call to McDonald's corporate HQ identifying myself as media requesting further explanation of the limited-time promotion resulted in no return call.
38. Reuters, "Wendy's Says Good-bye to Grapes," November 28, 2005.
39. Pressler, *Washington Post.*
40. For a detailed look at these issues, I highly recommend Eric Schlosser's *Fast Food Nation* (New York: Houghton Mifflin, 2001).

CHAPTER 5

1. Anthony Fletcher, "Food industry holds key to battling obesity," *Food Navigator*, July 25, 2005.
2. The guidelines are updated every five years. See "Key Recommendations" of the 2005 recommendations at: www.health.gov/dietaryguidelines/dga2005/recommendations.htm.
3. Kendall Powell, executive vice president, General Mills, remarks at the FTC Workshop "Perspectives on Marketing, Self-Regulation and Childhood Obesity," (July 14–15, 2005 Transcript available at www.ftc.gov/bcp/workshops/Foodmarketingtokids/transcript_050714.pdf.)
4. Marybeth Thorsgaard, telephone conversation with author, March 14, 2005.
5. Marion Nestle, e-mail message to author, March 16, 2005.
6. Fern Gale Estrow, telephone conversation with author, February 23, 2005.
7. Pauline Tinga, "Food Marketers Are Going 'PC,' " *Brand Packaging*, September 2005.
8. Margaret Webb Pressler, "Says Who? Food Companies Know What's Best. Just Ask Them," *Washington Post*, May 22, 2005.

9. Melinda Hemmelgarn, "Health Concerns Passing Convenience in Importance," *Columbia Daily Tribune*, March 16, 2005.

10. PepsiCo, press release, January 12, 2005, http://phx.corporate-ir.net/phoenix.zhtml?c=78265&p=irol-newsArticle&ID=662062&highlight=.

11. PepsiCo Web site, company overview. www.pepsico.com/PEP_Company/Overview/index.cfm.

12. Hoover's Web Site: http://www.hoovers.com/free/co/factsheet.xhtml?ID=48009.

13. PepsiCo, news release, April 15, 2004. http://phx.corporate-ir.net/phoenix.zhtml?c=78265&p=irol-newsArticle&ID=514833&highlight=.

14. Chad Terhune, "Pepsi Outlines Ad Campaign for Healthy Food," *Wall Street Journal*, October 25, 2005.

15. Ellen Taaffe, M.S., PepsiCo's vice president, Health and Wellness Marketing, "Presentation for the Workshop on Marketing Strategies that Foster Healthy Food and Beverage Choices in Children and Youth," January 27, 2005, available at: www.iom.edu/?id=24731.

16. Ibid.

17. Ibid.

18. Ibid.

19. Sarah Ellison, "Suit Challenges 'Low-Sugar' Cereals," *Wall Street Journal*, March 28, 2005.

20. "Montreal Woman Launches Suit against Kellogg," *Just-food.com*, June 21, 2005, www.just-food.com/news_detail.asp?art=61080.

21. Estrow, conversation.

22. Ira Teinowitz and Kate MacArthur, "McDonald's Ads Targets Children as Young as 4," *Ad Age*, January 28, 2005.

23. PepsiCo, annual report to investors, "Sustainable Advantage," 2004, p. 5. www.pepsico.com/PEP_Investors/AnnualReports/04/247528PepsicoLR.pdf.

24. Evelyn Ellison Twitchell, "Pepsi's Challenge," *SmartMoney*, December 14, 2005. http://www.smartmoney.com/mag/ceo/index.cfm?story=january2005.

25. Adrienne Carter, "Slimmer Kids, Fatter Profits?" *BusinessWeek*, September 5, 2005.

26. Jennifer Barrett Ozols, "Figuring Out the Labels," *Newsweek* (Web edition), March 15, 2005. http://msnbc.msn.com/id/7184067/site/newsweek/.

27. Renu Mansukhani, telephone conversation with author, February 19, 2006.

28. Kraft Web site: www.kraftfoods.com/kf/HealthyLiving/SensibleSolutions/CookiesAndCrackers.htm.

29. Mansukhani, conversation.

30. Melinda Hemmelgarn, e-mail message to author, March 14, 2005.

31. Sarah Ellison, "Why Kraft Decided to Ban Some Food Ads to Children," *Wall Street Journal*, November 1, 2005.

32. PowerAde Web site: www.us.powerade.com/advance/.

33. Coca-Cola Web site: www2.coca-cola.com/makeeverydropcount/hydration.html.
34. "Dehydration," *Teens Health.* http://kidshealth.org/teen/safety/first_aid/dehydration.html.
35. Ellison, "Why Kraft Decided to Ban Some Food Ads to Children."
36. Michael Bergeron (investigator) e-mail message to author that contained study results, as presented at the annual meeting of the American College of Sports Medicine but unpublished at press time.
37. Mansukhani, conversation.

CHAPTER 6

1. Kraft Foods Web site:
   www.kraftbrands.com/lunchables/index.aspx?area=game&SiteGameID=5014&RelationID=35.
2. Marion Nestle, *Food Politics* (Berkeley: University of California Press, 2002), 177–78.
3. See e.g., Susan Linn, *Consuming Kids* (New York: The New Press, 2004); Center for Science in the Public Interest, "Pestering Parents: How Food Companies Market Obesity to Children," November 2003. www.cspinet.org/new/200311101.html.
4. University of Illinois at Urbana-Champaign, press release, "TV Confuses Children about Which Foods Are Healthy, New Study Finds," June 6, 2005. www.news.uiuc.edu/news/05/0606kidfood.html.
5. Ibid.
6. General Mills, news release, June 6, 2005, at: www.generalmills.com/corporate/media_center/news_release_detail.aspx?itemID=11144&catID=227.
7. Julie Forster, "General Mills Ads Urge Kids to Eat Breakfast," *Pioneer Press*, June 23, 2005.
8. Ibid.
9. Ellen Fried, telephone conversation with author, August 11, 2005.
10. General Mills press release.
11. Fried, conversation.
12. Coca-Cola, press release, "The Coca-Cola Company's New Global Advertising and Promotion Policy for Children," July 15, 2003 http://www.coca-colahbc.com/cms/view.php?dir_pk=10&cms_pk=256.
13. In 2004, *American Idol* occupied twenty-three spots among the top-thirty viewed telecasts among kids two to eleven; even more astonishing, the January 28, 2004 telecast was the third most-viewed telecast (of any show) among kids two to eleven for the calendar year. www.nielsenmedia.com/newsreleases/2005/AmericanIdol2005.htm.
14. Theresa Howard, "Real Winner of *American Idol*: Coke," *USA Today*, September 8, 2002.
15. Coca-Cola press release.
16. Ibid.
17. Coca-Cola, "Model Guidelines for School Beverage Partnerships," http://www.corpschoolpartners.org/pdf/hal_school_beverage_guidelines.pdf.

18. Carolyn Dennis, telephone conversation with author, March 13, 2005.
19. Kraft Foods, press release, January 12, 2005. http://164.109.46.215/news-room/01122005.html.
20. See e.g., Dani Veracity, "Aspartame Promotes Grand Mal Seizures, Say Health Experts," *News Target*, June 27, 2005. www.newstarget.com/008952.html.
21. Renu Mansukhani, telephone conversation with author, February 19, 2006.
22. Mansukhani, conversation.
23. Adrienne Carter, "Slimmer Kids, Fatter Profits?" *BusinessWeek*, September 5, 2005, www.businessweek.com/magazine/content/05_36/b3949101.htm.
24. Kraft press release, January 12, 2005.
25. David Kiley, "SpongeBob: For Obesity or Health?" *BusinessWeek*, February 17, 2005.
26. John Consoli and Megan Larson, "Kids Upfront Gets Healthy," *MediaWeek*, February 21, 2005.
27. Kraft Foods, press release, September 15, 2005. www.kraft.com/news-room/09152005.html.
28. Mark Berlind, conversation with author, September 15, 2005.
29. Kraft Foods Web site: www.kraft.com/100/innovations/web.html.
30. Kraft Foods Web site: www.kraftbrands.com/lunchables/index.aspx?area=JMB_MISSION.
31. CARU Final Lunchables Decision, November 16, 2005. http://www.nadreview.org/LatestCaru.asp?SessionID=901046.
32. Ibid.
33. Kraft Foods Web site: www.kraftfoods.com/kf/HealthyLiving/SensibleSolutions/ConvenientMealProducts.htm.
34. Kraft Foods Web page on "Responsibility." www.kraft.com/responsibility/nhw_marketingpractices.aspx.
35. Caroline E. Mayer, "Kraft to Curb Snack-Food Advertising," *Washington Post*, January 12, 2005.
36. Mansukhani, conversation.
37. Delroy Alexander, "Kraft Will No Longer Aim Ads for Unhealthy Snacks at Youngsters," *Chicago Tribune*, January 13, 2005.
38. Editorial, "Kraft Takes Lead in Responsibility," *Advertising Age*, January 24, 2005.
39. Ben Hall, Dan Roberts, and Gary Silverman, "Obesity Fears Prompt Kraft to Stop Targeting Children with Junk Food Ads," Financial Times of London, January 13, 2005.
40. Sarah Ellison, "Why Kraft Decided to Ban Some Food Ads to Children," *Wall Street Journal*, November 1, 2005.
41. Sarah Ellison, "Divided, Companies Fight for Right to Plug Kids' Food," *Wall Street Journal*, January 26, 2005. PepsiCo later joined the coalition.
42. Susan Linn, e-mail message to author, March 19, 2005.
43. Gary Strauss, "Life's Good for SpongeBob," *USA Today*, May 17, 2002.
44. David Kiley, "SpongeBob: For Obesity or Health?" *BusinessWeek*, February 17, 2005.

45. Ibid.
46. Susan Linn, e-mail message to author, August 31, 2005.
47. See e.g., Juliet Schor's *Born to Buy* (New York: Scribner, 2004).

CHAPTER 7

1. Remarks by Tommy Thompson, U.S. secretary of health and human services, at the *Time*/ABC Summit on Obesity (June 2, 2004). (A webcast is available at www.rwjf.org.)
2. There are many ways that food companies influence government nutrition policies, but that is not my focus. See Marion Nestle's *Food Politics* for this side of the equation.
3. Teleconference hosted by Center for Science in the Public Interest, January 12, 2005.
4. Marion Nestle, e-mail message to author, January 13, 2005.
5. Remarks of Eric Bost, under secretary for food, nutrition and consumer services, U.S. Department of Agriculture, at "Food Guidance System Public Comment Meeting," August 19, 2004, Washington, D.C.
6. General Mills, press release, April 19, 2005. www.generalmills.com/corporate/ health_wellness/in_the_news_detail.aspx?itemID=10561&catID=7586&section=news.
7. Grocery Manufacturers Association, press release, April 19, 2005. www.gmabrands.com/news/docs/NewsRelease.cfm?DocID=1496.
8. Bost, remarks.
9. GMA press release, September 28, 2005. www.gmabrands.com/news/docs/ NewsRelease.cfm?DocID=1569.
10. U.S. Department of Health and Human Services, press release, March 9, 2004. www.hhs.gov/news/press/2004pres/20040309.html.
11. Center for Science in the Public Interest, press release, March 9, 2004. www.cspinet.org/new/200403092.html.
12. Daniel Yee, "Some Experts Say Cut Fat in Small Steps," *Associated Press*, March 10, 2004. www.phillyburbs.com/pb-dyn/news/248-03102004-262082.html.
13. "HHS Tackles Obesity," *FDA Consumer Magazine*, May–June 2004. www.fda.gov/fdac/features/2004/304_fat.html.
14. *Time*/ABC News Summit on Obesity. www.time.com/time/2004/obesity/.
15. Thompson, remarks, Summit.
16. Coca-Cola, "Model Guidelines for School Beverage Partnerships, 3 (2001) http://www.corpschoolpartners.org/pdf/hal_school_beverage_guidelines.pdf
17. Thompson, remarks, Summit on Obesity.
18. Niels Christensen, Nestlé; Betsy Holden, Kraft Foods; and Shelly Rosen, McDonald's, remarks at the *Time*/ABC Summit on Obesity, June 3, 2004.(A webcast is available at http://www.rwjf.org.)
19. Rosen, remarks, Summit.
20. Holden, remarks, Summit.
21. Carmona, remarks, Summit.

22. Ibid.

23. Susan Linn, e-mail message to author, July 20, 2005.

24. General Mills Web site: www.generalmills.com/corporate/commitment/champions.aspx.

25. Form 10-Q Filing for General Mills, January 6, 2006 http://biz.yahoo.com/e/060106/gis10-q.html.

26. President's Challenge Web site: www.presidentschallenge.org/advocates/corporate.aspx.

CHAPTER 8

1. Carol Hogan, at "Legal and Strategic Guide to Minimizing Liability for Obesity: What Food Industry Counsel Need to Know Now," Chicago, September 8, 2004. Hogan also advised that industry experts be believable, down-to-earth, and likable.

2. Terrence Gaffney, conversation with author, September 8, 2004.

3. Josh Golin, letter to the editor, *Journal of Nutrition Education and Behavior*, June 2005.

4. Liz Marr, "Soft Drinks, Childhood Overweight and the Role of Nutrition Educators: Let's Base Our Solutions on Reality and Sound Science," *Journal of Nutrition Education and Behavior*, September 2004, 262.

5. Josh Golin, letter.

6. Virginia Tech, press release, "Soft Drinks Not Linked to Decreased Calcium Intake," March 26, 2004. www.sciencedaily.com/releases/2004/03/040325071447.htm.

7. See e.g., "Liquid Candy," Center for Science in the Public Interest, 2005; teen boys who drink soda do so at the rate of 28.5 ounces per day; one-quarter of teen girls who drink soda down at least two cans per day.

8. See e.g., Jennifer Washburn, *University, Inc.: The Corporate Corruption of American Higher Education* (New York: Basic Books, 2005).

9. Carla Rivera, "Childhood Obesity Off the Scale in California," *Los Angeles Times*, September 9, 2005.

10. Rick Berman, "Soft Drink Hysteria Hard to Swallow," *Atlanta Journal-Constitution*, August 26, 2004.

11. ACFN Web site: http://www.acfn.org/about/.

12. ACFN Web site: http://www.acfn.org/a3/.

13. Susan Finn, "A Winning Recipe for Curbing Obesity," *Chicago Sun-Times*, November 27, 2003.

14. SourceWatch.org Web site: www.sourcewatch.org/index.php?title=ACSH. In their books *Toxic Sludge Is Good for You* and *Trust Us, We're Experts!*, authors John Stauber and Sheldon Rampton do an excellent job exposing ACSH's distortions and lies.

15. Elizabeth Whelan, "A Year of Public Health Lunacy," the *New York Post*, December 16, 2005. www.acsh.org/healthissues/newsID.1254/healthissue_detail.asp.

16. Melanie Warner, "Is a Trip to McDonald's Just What the Doctor Ordered?" the *New York Times*, May 2, 2005.

17. McDonald's Web site: www.mcdonalds.com/usa/eat/ornish.html.
18. Warner, *New York Times.*
19. Ibid.
20. Kraft Foods, press release, www.kraft.com/obesity/09032003.html.
21. American Diabetes Association, press release, April 21, 2005: www.diabetes.org/for-media/2005-press-releases/cadbury-schweppes.jsp.
22. Commercial Alert, press release, April 21, 2005: www.commercialalert.org/blog/archives/2005/04/index.html.
23. "Diabetes Association Defends Cadbury Schweppes Deal," *Corporate Crime Reporter* 209, May 16, 2005: www.corporatecrimereporter.com/diabetes051605.htm.
24. Ibid.
25. Russell Mokhiber and Robert Weissman, "Our Public Health Groups: All Fall Down," *CommonDreams.org*, May 16, 2005, at: www.commondreams.org/views05/0516-33.htm.
26. Bell Institute Web site: www.bellinstitute.com/bihn/about_us/index.aspx?cat_1=28.
27. General Mills, press release, March 22, 2005: www.bellinstitute.com/bihn/news/news_detail.aspx?cat_1=25&extCat ID=7586&extItemID=9715.
28. Jerry Markon, "Dairy Industry Sued Over Weight-Loss Claims," *Washington Post*, June 29, 2005. http://www.washingtonpost.com/wp-dyn/content/article/2005/06/28/AR2005062800834.html
29. "The Dairy Weight Loss Debate," *Tufts Health and Nutrition Letter*, September 2005. http://healthletter.tufts.edu/issues/2005-09/dairy.html.
30. Physicians Committee Responsible Medicine, press release, June 28, 2005: www.pcrm.org/cgi-bin/lists/mail.cgi?flavor=archive&id=20050628100850&list=news.
31. Kraft Foods Web site: "The Role of Dairy in Healthy Weight," www.kraftfoods.com/kf/HealthyLiving/DairyWeightManagement/DWM_art icle_DiscoveringtheRoleofDairyinHealthyWeight.htm.
32. The Beverage Institute for Health & Wellness, Mission and Scope. www.the-beverageinstitute.org/mission_scope.shtml.
33. See e.g., various press releases and fact sheets from the India Resource Center. www.indiaresource.org/.
34. Haider Rizvi, "Coke Slammed at Shareholders Meeting for Practices in India," *OneWorld.net*, April 21, 2006.
35. Diabetes India Association: www.diabetesindia.com/.
36. The Beverage Institute for Health & Wellness, Symposiums. www.thebeverage institute.org/symposiums.shtml.
37. Richard Daynard, e-mail message to author, March 19, 2005. For the results of the study, see David S. Ludwig, Karen E. Peterson, and Steven L. Gortmaker, "Relationship between Consumption of Sugar-Sweetened Drinks and Childhood Obesity," *The Lancet* 357 (2001): 505–508.

38. E-mail from Richard Daynard.

39. Ibid.

40. The Beverage Institute for Health & Wellness, Symposiums.

41. John N. Frank, "Oldways Gathering to Give Sugar Positive PR," *PR Week*, September 22, 2004. www.prweek.com/us/search/article/222977/old-ways-gathering-give-sugar-positive-pr.

42. Ibid.

43. "Oldways Develops Tools for Consumers to Manage Sweetness and Focus on the Total Diet Instead of 'Bits and Pieces,' " *PR Newswire*, November 10, 2004. www.prnewswire.com/cgi-bin/stories.pl?ACCT=104&STORY=/www/story/11-10-2004/0002402326&EDATE=.

44. Oldways Web site: http://oldwayspt.org/index.php?area=oldways_history.

45. The Coalition for a Healthy and Active America Web site: www.chaausa.org/index.asp?Type=B_EV&SEC={AE3C2468-896B-461E-B8AE-94A5962A8699.

CHAPTER 9

1. National Restaurant Association, "Nutrition/Menu Labeling Talking Points," available at: www.restaurant.org/government/state/nutrition/resources/nra_20040208_talkingpoints_labeling.pdf.

2. Marc Santora, "East Meets West: Adding Pounds and Peril," *New York Times*, January 12, 2006.

3. National Restaurant Association: www.restaurant.org/research/ind_glance.cfm.

4. CSPI, "Anyone's Guess: The Need for Nutrition Labeling at Fast-Food and Other Chain Restaurants," November 2003. www.cspinet.org/restaurantreport.pdf.

5. USDA Factbook, Chapter 2, "Profiling Food Consumption in America." www.usda.gov/factbook/chapter2.pdf.

6. "AC Nielsen Finds U.S. Truly Is a Fast Food Nation," December 21, 2004 http://us.acnielsen.com/news/20041221.shtml.

7. C. Zoumas-Morse, C. L. Rock, E. J. Sobo, and M. L. Newhouser. "Children's Patterns of Macronutrient Intake and Associations with Restaurant and Home Eating." *Journal of the American Dietetic Association* 101 (2001): 923–25.

8. National Restaurant Association "At a Glance." www.restaurant.org/research/ind_glance.cfm.

9. CSPI, "Anyone's Guess."

10. Ibid.

11. National Restaurant Association, "Nutrition/Menu Labeling Talking Points."

12. Terrence Dopp, "Lawmakers Want Restaurant Chains to Count Calories," *NJ.com*, February 13, 2005. www.nj.com/news/sunbeam/index.ssf?/base/news-2/1107422416165050.xml.

13. CSPI, "Anyone's Guess."

14. Ellen Fried, e-mail message to author, October 31, 2005.

15. Sean Faircloth, telephone conversation with author, March 28, 2005.

16. Ibid.
17. McDonald's, press release, October 25, 2005. www.mcdonalds.com/corp/ news/corppr/2005/cpr_10252005.html.
18. Letter from McDonald's to U.S. Food and Drug Administration, April 18, 1975. (Emphasis in original.)
19. Stephen Gardner, telephone conversation with author, February 13, 2006.
20. Ibid.
21. Ibid.
22. Richard E. Marriott, "FDA Fresh Labeling Regulations Go 'Light' on Menus: Food and Drug Administration Exempts Restaurant Menus from Regulations," *Nation's Restaurant News*, March 15, 1993.
23. Marc Santora, *New York Times*.
24. Felix Ortiz, telephone conversation with author, January 30, 2006.
25. Robert Stern, telephone conversation with author, February 1, 2006.
26. Ibid.
27. Record of Proceedings, The Assembly of the State of New York, June 22, 2005.
28. Ibid.
29. Ortiz, conversation.
30. Faircloth, conversation.
31. Ibid.
32. Ibid.
33. Dorsey Griffith, "Food Industry Puts Its Weight into Obesity Fight," *Sacramento Bee*, May 24, 2004.
34. Ibid.
35. Phil Mendelson, telephone conversation with author, January 23, 2006.
36. "Commonsense Compromise Rejected by Food Industry," blog posting, May 11, 2005. www.phaionline.org/weblog/archives/2005/05/index.php.
37. Associated Press, "Bill Preventing Obesity Lawsuits Stuck in Subcommittee," March 15, 2006, www.myrtlebeachonline.com/mld/ myrtlebeachonline/news/local.
38. Jon Olinto, e-mail message to author, October 29, 2005.
39. Ben Kelley, e-mail message to author, October 26, 2005.

CHAPTER 10

1. Scott Leith, "A Push to Stay in Schools: A Target of Anti-Sugar Activists, CCE Defends Its Sales in Schools," *Atlanta Journal-Constitution*, March 6, 2003.
2. Marion Nestle, *Food Politics* and Kelly Brownell, *Food Fight*.
3. United States General Accounting Office, *School Lunch Program: Efforts Needed to Improve Nutrition and Encourage Healthy Eating*. GAO report number 03-056, Washington, D.C., 2003.
4. CSPI, "Dispensing Junk: How School Vending Undermines Efforts to Feed Children Well," May 2004. http://cspinet.org/new/pdf/dispensing_ junk.pdf. (The percentage should be higher since researchers counted diet drinks in the "healthy" category.)

5. *National Soft Drink Association v. Block*, 721 F.2d 1348 (D.C. Cir. 1983).

6. Jacqueline Domac, telephone conversation with author, August 30, 2004.

7. Deborah Ortiz, telephone conversation with author, August 30, 2004.

8. Ibid.

9. Domac, telephone conversation.

10. Carolyn Dennis, telephone conversation with author, March 13, 2005.

11. Ibid.

12. Ibid.

13. Sullivan & LeShane, Government Relations Welcome Page, www.ctlobby.com/govrelations/html/indexre.htm (citing the *Hartford Courant*). Last visited September 20, 2005.

14. Gregory B. Hladky, "Soda Makers Pull Out All Stops to Put Big Chill on School Ban," *Bristol Press*, May 7, 2005.

15. Dailykos.com, "CT Gov. Rell Kowtows to Big Cola on Junk Food," www.dailykos.com/storyonly/2005/7/30/112038/037.

16. Alison Leigh Cowan, "Healthy Food in the Lunchroom? First, You Need a Healthy Debate," *New York Times*, May 16, 2005.

17. Sullivan & LeShane, Government Relations, firm bios, Patricia "Paddi" LeShane, www.ctlobby.com/shared/bios/b-patricia.html.

18. Patricia LeShane contributed a total of $1,300 to the 2002 Connecticut gubernatorial campaign. Followthemoney.org, State at a Glance: Connecticut 2002, Contributors, LeShane, Patricia,: http://www.followthemoney.org/database/StateGlance/contributor.phtml?si=20027&d=4533548.

19. Lucy Nolan, e-mail message to author, March 9, 2006.

20. Thomas Farley, e-mail message to author, July 5, 2005.

21. New Mexico School Nutrition Committee Considers Vending Restrictions, July 15th, 2005. http://www.amonline.com/article/article.jsp?id=14232&siteSection=1.

22. Editorial, "Junk Food Jitterbug: Vicki Walker Dances Away from Tougher Rules," *The Register-Guard* (Eugene, Oregon), May 16, 2005.

23. Joy Johanson, telephone conversation with author, March 19, 2005.

24. Brita Butler-Wall, telephone conversation with author, August, 23 2004.

25. Kari Bjorhus, telephone conversation with author, August 25, 2004.

26. Michael Butler, telephone conversation with author, August 17, 2004.

27. Sean Faircloth, telephone conversation with author, July 9, 2004.

28. Community Health Partnership, School Soda Contracts: A Sample Review of Contracts in Oregon Public School Districts, 2004. http://www.communityhealthpartnership.org/publications/reports/soda_contracts/soda_report/soda_summary.html

29. Bjorhus, telephone conversation.

30. Brett McFadden, telephone conversation with author, August 20, 2004.

31. Butler, telephone conversation.

32. Dennis, telephone conversation.

33. "Kelly's War on Junk Food," *The Guardian*, September 29, 2005.

CHAPTER 11

1. Jonathan Eig, "Edible Entertainment—Food Companies Grab Kids by Fancifully Packaging Products as Toys, Games," *Wall Street Journal*, October 24, 2001.

2. CSPI, "Pestering Parents: How Food Companies Market Obesity to Children," November 2003. www.cspinet.org/new/200311101.html: see also Susan Linn, *Consuming Kids*.

3. American Psychological Association, "Report of the APA Task Force on Advertising and Children," February 20, 2004, available at www.apa.org/releases/childrenads_summary.pdf.

4. Susan Linn and Josh Golin, "Beyond Commercials: How Food Marketers Target Children," 39 *Loy. Of L.A. Law Rev.* 13 (2006).

5. Live symposium, "Food Marketing to Children and the Law," Loyola Law School, Los Angeles, October 21, 2005. To view the video presentations, visit: www.informedeating.org/newsletters/051115.htm.

6. Institute of Medicine, "Food Marketing to Children and Youth: Threat or Opportunity?" December 6, 2005. www.iom.edu/?id=31330&redirect=0.

7. Ellen Wartella, speaking at Institute of Medicine public briefing, "Food Marketing to Children and Youth," December 6, 2005; audio available at: www.iom.edu/?id=31330&redirect=0.

8. Linn, *Consuming Kids*, 147.

9. Remarks by Senator Tom Harkin (D-IA) at the FTC/HHS workshop "Perspectives on Marketing, Self-Regulation and Childhood Obesity," July 13, 2005, http://harkin.senate.gov/news.cfm?id=240635.

10. Ellen Fried, e-mail message to author, March 23, 2006.

11. Tracy Westen, "Government Regulation of Food Marketing to Children: The Federal Trade Commission and the Kid-Vid Controversy," 39, *Loy. Of L.A. Law Rev.* 79 (2006).

12. Ibid.

13. Ibid.

14. Dan Jaffe, Association of National Advertisers, remarks as quoted in: http://promomagazine.com/news/institute_medicine_study_120705/

15. Debora Platt-Majoras, Commissioner, Federal Trade Commission, Remarks at the FTC/HHS workshop, "Perspectives on Marketing, Self-Regulation and Childhood Obesity," July 14—15, 2005, transcript day one, available at: www.ftc.gov/bcp/workshops/foodmarketingtokids/transcript_050714.pdf.

16. Tracy Westen, 11

17. Angela Campbell, "Restricting the Marketing of Junk Food to Children by Product Placement and Character Selling," 39 *Loy. Of L.A. Law Rev.* 447 (2006).

18. Marion Nestle, remarks at the *Time*/ABC Summit on Obesity (June 3, 2004). (A webcast is available at http://www.rwjf.org.)

19. Institute of Medicine report.

20. See Marion Nestle, *Food Politics*, 131.

21. Remarks of Tommy Thompson, U.S. Secretary of Health and Human Services,

at the *Time*/ABC Summit on Obesity (June 2, 2004). (A webcast is available at http://www.rwjf.org.)

22. Stephen Gardener, "Litigation as a Tool in Food Advertising: A Consumer Advocacy Viewpoint," 39 *Loy. Of L.A. Law Rev.* 291 (2006).

23. CSPI press release, January 18, 2006. www.cspinet.org/new/200601181.html.

24. Remarks of Richard Carmona, surgeon general, at FTC/HHS Workshop, "Perspectives on Marketing, Self-Regulation and Childhood Obesity," July 14—15, 2005, transcript day two. www.ftc.gov/bcp/workshops/foodmarketingtokids/transcript_050715.pdf.

25. Margo Wootan, director of nutrition policy, CSPI, remarks at FTC/HHS Workshop, "Perspectives on Marketing, Self-Regulation and Childhood Obesity," July 14–15, 2005, transcript day two. www.ftc.gov/bcp/workshops/foodmarketingtokids/transcript_050715.pdf.

26. Thanks to the Campaign for a Commercial-Free Childhood for some of these ideas.

27. Senator Harkin remarks, FTC/HHS Workshop.

28. Juliet Schor, *Born to Buy* (New York: Scribner, 2004).

29. Corinna Hawkes, "Marketing Food to Children: The Global Regulatory Environment," World Health Organization, 2004. http://whqlibdoc.who.int/publications/2004/9241591579.pdf

30. Institute of Medicine report.

31. Ibid.

32. Radley Balko, "Food for Thought on Childhood Obesity," *Foxnews.com*, February 21, 2005. www.foxnews.com/story/0,2933,148208,00.html.

33. Neville Rigby, e-mail message to author, February 10, 2006.

34. Corinna Hawkes, e-mail message to author, February 10, 2006.

35. The World Bank, "Curbing the Epidemic: Governments and the Economics of Tobacco Control," 1999. http://www1.worldbank.org/tobacco/reports.asp

36. Senator Thomas Harkin, press release, "Harkin Pushes Comprehensive Wellness Initiative to Fight Chronic Disease, Obesity and Reduce Health Care Costs" (May 18, 2005). http://harkin.senate.gov/news.cfm?id=237846.

37. These ideas and more like them can be found in. Randolph Kline, Samantha Graff, Leslie Zellers, and Marice Ashe, "Beyond Advertising Controls: Influencing Junk-Food Marketing and Consumption with Policy Innovations Developed in Tobacco Control", 39 *Loy. Of L.A. Law Rev.* 603 (2006)

CHAPTER 12

1. Press release, Wisconsin's Governor's Office, March 17, 2004. www.wisgov.state.wi.us/journal_media_detail.asp?prid=443.

2. Marc Santora, "Teenagers' Suit Says McDonald's Made Them Obese," *New York Times*, November 21, 2002.

3. Bryan Malenius, telephone conversation with author, March 1, 2005.

4. Press release, Wisconsin's Governor's Office, March 17, 2004. Sadly, this same

governor signed a similar bill in 2006, explaining that the difference now was that "other states" were doing it.

5. *Ashley Pelman v. McDonald's Corp.*, 237 F. Supp.2d 512 (S.D.N.Y. Jan. 22, 2003).

6. Ibid.

7. Ellen Fried, telephone conversation with author, February 27, 2005.

8. Mindy Kursban, telephone conversation with author, February 26, 2005.

9. University of California, San Francisco, Legacy Tobacco Documents Library. http://legacy.library.ucsf.edu/.

10. Neal Barnard, *Breaking the Food Seduction* (New York: St. Martin's Press, 2003).

11. Dr. William Jacobs of the University of Florida speaking at the Second Annual Conference on Legal Strategies in the Obesity Epidemic, September 2004.

12. Malenius, conversation.

13. National Restaurant Association Web site. www.restaurant.org/government/state/nutrition/bills_lawsuits.cfm#overview.

14. National Restaurant Association Web site. www.restaurant.org/government/state/nutrition/resources.cfm.

15. Fried, conversation.

16. Center for Consumer Freedom Web site. www.consumerfreedom.com/advertisements_detail.cfm/ad/6.

17. "Houston Bill Cuts Eatery Exposure," *Contra Costa Times*, March 4, 2005.

18. John Dutra testifying at California Assembly Committee on judiciary bill hearing, May 4, 2004.

19. Ibid.

CHAPTER 13

1. Tim Longhurst, "Progressive Quotes," November 17, 2005. www.timlonghurst.com/content/view/98/48/.

2. Kelly Brownell, *Time*/ABC News Summit on Obesity, Williamsburg, June 3, 2004.

3. Richard Daynard, telephone conversation with author, February 19, 2006.

4. Sean Faircloth, telephone conversation with author, March 28, 2005.

5. Juliet Schor, *Born to Buy*.

6. Carol McGruder, "Tobacco's Global Ghettos: Big Tobacco Targets the World's Poor," CorpWatch, June 30, 1997. www.corpwatch.org/article.php?id=3970.

7. Yum! Brands Web site: www.yum.com/investors/default.asp.

8. The Global Spread of Food Uniformity, Worldwatch Institute. www.worldwatch.org/pubs/goodstuff/fastfood/.

9. Reuters, "McDonald's Opening Drive-Thru Windows in China," January 12, 2006. www.foxnews.com/story/0,2933,181468,00.html.

10. Coca-Cola Web site: www2.coca-cola.com/ourcompany/aroundworld.html.

11. "Interesting India," *Financial Times*, March 31, 2005.

12. PepsiCo, 2005 annual report. http://ccbn.mobular.net/ccbn/7/1250/1337/print/print.pdf.

13. Helena Norberg-Hodge, Todd Merrifield, and Steven Gorelick, *Bringing the Food Economy Home: Local Alternatives to Global Agribusiness*, (Bloomfield, CT: Kumarian Press, 2002) 30–31.
14. Richard Ganis, "Food Fight: Rethinking Approaches to Sustainable Agriculture," *Wild Matters*, September 2002. www.usenet.com/newsgroups/misc.activism.progressive/msg05294.html

INDEX

5 a Day program, xvii, 27, 260
80-20 rule, 80–81

A
ABC News, 156
access to healthy food, 25–26
Active Achievers program, 35
activist judges, 323
ActivistCash, 52–53
Advance, 110
advergaming, 117, 129–30, 248–49, 323
advertising. *See* marketing
African American community, 77
Agribusiness Accountability Initiative, 359
Allen, Lee, 5, 7–9
Allen, Sandy, 212
Alliance for American Advertising, 135, 332
Alm, John, 219
Altria, 124
America on the Move, 160, 336
American Advertising Federation, 332
American Association of Advertising Agencies, 135, 332
American Beverage Association (ABA), 13–19, 29, 171, 331
American Cancer Society, 305
American Council on Fitness and Nutrition (ACFN), xxi, 176–78, 333
American Council on Science and Health (ACSH), 178–79, 333
American Diabetes Association (ADA), 182–86
American Dietetic Association (ADA), 176
American Heart Association (AHA), 17
American Idol, 122, 248, 250
American Legislative Exchange Council, 333
American Lung Association, 305
American Tort Reform Association, 333
America's Walking, 153
Anderson, Steven, 22
Apple Dippers, 74–75
Applebee's International, 64
Arizona schools, 234
Armstrong, Lance, 37–38
artificial foods, xii
aspartame, 126
Association of California School Administrators (ACSA), 239
Association of National Advertisers, 332
astroturf campaigns, 323
Atlanta Journal-Constitution, 15, 175

Au Bon Pain, 72
Austin, Denise, 147

B
Bacon, Linda, 32
Bakan, Joel, 3, 10–11
Balance First program, 38, 334
Balanced, Active Lifestyles initiative, 72
balanced diet, 323
Balanced for Life, 334
Balanced Lifestyles Platform, 153
Barnard, Neal, 47
Beall, Sandy, 11
Bell Institute of Health and Nutrition, 186, 334
Berlind, Mark, 129, 132
Berman, Richard, 45–47, 60, 62–64, 175
better-for-you products, 323
Beverage Institute for Health & Wellness, 188, 334
b.good restaurant, 214–16
"Big Food Lawsuits Can Help Trim America's Waistline", 284–85
Bittler, David, 137
Bjorhus, Kari, 237, 239
Blackburn, George, 181
Blair, Tony, 240
blame, 42–43
Blue Ribbon Advisory Board, 180, 334
Born to Buy, 264, 308
Bradley, Israel, 274
Bradley, Jazlyn, 273, 277
brand licensing, 248
brand loyalty, 323–24
Brand New You program, 335
branded playgrounds, 33–34

British schools, 240–41
Brock, Rovenia, 76–77
Brown, Charlie, xix, 153, 234
Brownell, Kelly, 302
Burger King, 9, 79–80
Burton, Bob, 63
Bush, George W., 203–4
Butler, Michael, 237, 239
Butler-Wall, Brita, 236
Buyckx, Maxime, 189–90
buzz, 324

C
Cadbury Schweppes, 182–86
caffeine, 110
calcium, 171
California
    clean air act, 270
    legislation, 293–95
    schools, 242
    soda ban, 224–26
California Center for Public Health Advocacy (CCPHA), 225, 294, 357
California Food and Justice Coalition, 357
California Project LEAN, 357
callouts, 324
caloric intake, xiii, 342
Camargo, Carlos, 145
Campaign for a Commercial-Free Childhood (CCFC), 36, 170, 247, 260–61, 355
Campbell, Angela, 258
Campbell's Center for Nutrition and Wellness, 334
Canada, 266
Capri-Sun Sport drink, 110–11
carbohydrates, 93
cardiovascular disease, xiv

Carmona, Richard, 154–56, 262
cartoons, 130–31, 138–39, 258
celebrity endorsements, 75–78
Center for Consumer Freedom
  (CCF)
  corporate donations, 66
  litigation, 290–93
  menu labeling, 211–12
  obesity, 172–76
  soda bans, 225
  tactics, xxi, 23–24, 30, 46–66
  web site, 333
Center for Food and Nutrition
  Policy (CENP), 171
Center for Informed Food
  Choices, 47, 355
Center for Media and Democracy,
  62–64, 360
Center for Public Integrity, 360
Center for Responsive Politics, 360
Center for Science in the Public
  Interest (CSPI), xxii, 51, 196,
  198, 204, 247, 260, 355
Centers for Disease Control and
  Prevention (CDC), 175
cereals, 94–97, 104–5
Champions for Healthy Kids, 336
character merchandising, 324
check mark icons, 105
cheeseburger bills, 289, 324
cheese, xii
Chicken McNugget ingredients, 280
"The Childhood Obesity Epidemic: Predictors and Strategies
  for Prevention", 189
children
  marketing to, 117–42, 245–71
  obesity, xv, 307–8
  schools, 219–44
  television, 250–51

Children's Advertising Review
  Unit (CARU), 119–21, 130,
  251–52, 332
China, 309–10
choice, 324
CHOICE: Citizens for Healthy
  Options in Children's Educa-
  tion, 355
Choose Breakfast campaign,
  120–21
Christensen, Niels, 154
Citizens for Responsibility and
  Ethics in Washington (CREW),
  61–62
Clinton, Bill, 17–18, 22
Clinton Foundation, 17
Coalition for a Healthy and Active
  America, 336
Coalition for Healthy Children,
  336
Coalition of Immokalee Workers,
  358
cobranding, 324
Coca-Cola Company
  CCF contributions, 64
  education, 37–42
  marketing to children, xix, 18,
    121–23, 152–54, 169–70,
    220–44
  research, 188–91
  sports drinks, 110
Commercial Alert, xxii, 183, 247,
  309, 355
commercial speech, 256–57
commitment, 324
Commonsense Consumption Act,
  274, 289
communication, 324
Community Food Security Coalition, 356

complex carbohydrates, 93
complex issue, 325
compromise, 313
Connecticut schools, 231–33
consumer freedom, 50
ConsumerDeception.com, 360
Consuming Kids, 35, 135, 158, 248
convenience, 325
Corporate Accountability Project, 361
Corporate Crime Reporter (CCR), 184
The Corporation, 3, 10–11
corporations, 2–19
    brand imaging, xv
    responsibility, 325
Council for Corporate and School Partnerships, 333
Crist, Paul, 284–85
cross promotions, 248, 325
CSPIscam, 51

D
diary industry, 187–88
Daynard, Richard, 42–43, 64, 190, 268, 303
D.C. Public Schools (DCPS), 236
Dean Foods Company, 64
dehydration, 109
Dennis, Carolyn, 228–30, 239, 343–45
Department of Health and Human Services (HHS), 150
Deromedi, Roger, 125
Destiny's Child, 76–77
developing countries, 309–11
diabetes, 182–86, 189
Dietary Guidelines for Americans, 144

Dillon, Mary, 72
disease foundations, 182–86
Dollins, Mark, 34
Domac, Jacqueline, 227–28
Dooley, Cal, 91
Doyle, Jim, 273, 277
Dutra, John, 293–94

E
Easterbrook, Frank H., 3
eating out, 195–217
education, xvii, xxii, 37–42
energy balance, 29–36, 148–49, 161, 325
Estrow, Fern Gale, 96, 105
Excel/Cargill, 64
exclusive contracting, 325
exercise, 29–36, 308
externalizing costs, 7

F
failure to disclose, 279–80
Faircloth, Sean, 200, 210–11, 238, 304, 343
Fairly OddParents, 131
farm-to-school program, 315
fast food, 67–89
    economics of, 81–87
    healthier products, 85–89
    nutrition labeling, 339–42
    press releases, 88–89
Fast Food Nation, 24
fat, xi, xiii
federal agencies, 57
Federal Communications Commission (FCC), 249–50
Federal Trade Commission (FTC), 156–58, 250, 252–53
Feed Me Better Campaign, 241, 359

Fenton, Mark, 153
Finn, Susan, 31, 176–78
First Amendment, 255–58
Fishel, Daniel R., 3
Fit It In program, 335
Florio, Dale, 199
food addictions, 283
Food and Drug Administration
    (FDA), 151
Food Commission, 359
Food First, 359
Food Guide Pyramid, 146–50
The Food Institute Daily Update, 337
food police, 50, 54, 325
Food Policy Blog, 358
Food Politics, 53, 95–96, 120, 145,
    161, 258
Food Products Association (FPA),
    285–86, 331
The Food Project, 358
food pyramid, 94, 146–50
Food Secure Canada, 359
The Food Studies Institute, 356
The Food Trust, 358
Ford, Sabrina, 78
free speech, 255–59, 325
freedom of choice, 22, 326
Freedom of Information Center,
    361
french fries, 69–70
Fried, Ellen, 121, 200, 252, 281,
    289
Friedman, Lance, 107
Friedman, Milton, 4
Frito-Lay, 92, 101
frivolous lawsuits, 326, 330
Frommer, Dario, 227
fruits, xii, 144
fun-for-you products, 326
functional benefit, 326

G
Gaffney, Bennett & Associates,
    231
Gaffney, Terrence, 168
Gardner, Stephen, 202, 260–61
Gatorade, 101, 109
Gatorade Sports Science Institute,
    334
General Mills
    cereal, 94–98, 104–5, 148
    marketing to children, 135, 159
    public relations, 9, 92, 120–21,
        159
    yogurt, 187
Get Active Stay Active program,
    335
Get Fit Challenge, 335
Get Kids in Action, 336
Gillespie, Ray, 229
Girls on the Run, 335
Global Advisory Council on Bal-
    anced Lifestyles, 180, 334
globalization, 309–11
GM Watch, 359
Go Active! Adult Happy Meal,
    83–84
Goldstein, Harold, 294
Golin, Josh, 170
good-for-you products, 326
Gottfried, Richard, 208
government, 57
    complicity, 143–65
    lobbying, 326
GRACE Factory Farm Project,
    356
green color, 100, 105
Greenburg, Danielle, 235
greenwashing, 67–68
Grocery Manufacturers Association
    (GMA), xx, 25, 135

food pyramid, 149
school policy, 223–24
soft drinks, 210, 230, 234
web site, 331
the growth imperative, 5
Guest Choice Network, 46

H

halo effect, 71, 75–78, 81, 84, 326
Happy Meals, 74–75
Harkin, Tom, 251, 263, 269
Harrison, Kristen, 119
Haugen, John, 148
Hawkes, Corinna, 268
health advisors, 179–82
Health and Human Services
    (HHS), 71
Health Care Without Harm, 356
health organizations, 182–86
healthy lifestyles, 326–27
Healthy Lifestyles and Disease Pre-
    vention Initiative, 150
Healthy Lifestyles and Prevention
    (HeLP) America Act, 269
heavy users, 327
Hemmelgarn, Melinda, 99–100,
    110
Hershey Center for Health and
    Nutrition, 334
high blood pressure, xiii
high schools, 226–28
    See also schools
hip-hop, 77–78
Hispanic community, 149–50
Hogan, Carol, 167
Holden, Betsy, 154
host selling, 250, 327
human evolution, xi
hunter-gatherer cultures, xiii
hydration, 327

I

in-store promotions, 327
India, 189
India Resource Center, 359–60
Indiana schools, 234
individual choice, xvii
industry groups, 331–37
initiative, 327
Institute for Agriculture and Trade
    Policy, 356
Institute of Medicine (IOM),
    101–3, 124, 249–50, 255–56,
    259
The Institute on Money in State
    Politics, 361
interactive product placement, 327
International Food Information
    Council, 333
International Food Policy
    Research Institute, 360
International Journal of Obesity,
    187
International Life Sciences Insti-
    tute, 334
International Obesity Taskforce,
    267
internet advertising, 129–30
Isdell, E. Neville, 170

J

Jacobson, Michael F., 51, 204
Jaffe, Dan, 255
Johanns, Mike, 147
Jones Day, 284
Joseph, Stephen, 70
*Journal of Nutrition Education
    and Behavior (JNEB)*, 169
*Journal of the American Medical
    Association (JAMA)*, 175
junk culture, 308

junk science, 51, 327
Just Food, 358

K

Kahn, Richard, 184–86
Keller, Ric, 22, 276, 287, 296
Kelley, Ben, 214–15
Kellogg, 9, 105, 135, 260
Kelly, Petra, 299
Kelly, Ruth, 241
Kentucky schools, 228–31
Kessler, David, 180
Kid Power conference, 264
Kid-Vid initiative, 252
Kidnetic.com, 335
Kiley, David, 77–78, 128, 137
Kraft Foods
    dairy products, 188
    logos, 99–100, 105
    Lunchables, 126–27, 130,
        133–34
    marketing to children, 123–36
    portion control, 97
    public relations, 9, 92, 181
    Sensible Solutions program,
        107–10
Kretser, Alison, 31, 41–42
Kroc, Ray, 67, 81
Kursban, Mindy, 282

L

labeling, 98–100, 195–217,
    339–42
Lascoutx, Elizabeth, 121
lawsuits, 260–61, 273–98, 325
    frivolous, 288–89
Leach, Brock, 33–34
Leary, Thomas, 156
Ledbetter, Sam, 213
"Legal and Strategic Guide to

Minimizing Liability for Obesity
    Conference: What Food
    Industry @index:Counsel Need
    to Know Now", 284
legal rights, 273–98, 351–54
LeShane, Patricia, 233
licensing, 327
Linn, Susan, 35–36, 135, 138,
    158, 245, 248–49
liquid candy, 184, 188
litigation, 260–61, 273–98, 325
Live It! program, 38–39, 335
local control, 327–28
Lorillard v. Reilly, 257
Los Angeles Unified School District, 224–25, 227–28
Louisiana schools, 234–35
Ludwig, David, 110
Lunchables, 126–27, 130, 133–34

M

Majoras, Deborah Platt, 256
Malcynsky, Jay F., 231
Malenius, Bryan, 276, 287
Managing Sweetness conference,
    190
Mander, Jerry, 6
Mansukhani, Renu, 108–9, 111,
    126–27, 134
marketing, 27
    to children, 117–42, 245–71
    health-themed, 91
"Marketing, Self-Regulation, and
    Childhood Obesity", 156
Marr Barr Communications, 169
Marr, Liz, 169–70
Massachusetts Public Health Association, 358
McDonald's, 9, 67–89, 180
    corporate mascot, 34–36

globalization, 310–11
Happy Meals, 74–75
healthier products, 85–88,
    152–53
lawsuits, 273–81, 296
nutrition labeling, 200–205,
    215–16
salads, 72–74, 82–85
trans fat, 12, 70–71
McFadden, Brett, 239
McGrievy, Brie Turner, 73
McLibel case, 296
Mendelson, Phil, 212–13
Miller, James, 254
Mindus, Dan, 30, 173–74
moderation, 328
Mokhiber, Russell, 185
moms, 328
movie tie-ins, 248
MyPyramid, 94, 146–50, 162

N
Nabisco, 97
Nader, Ralph, 254
nag factor, 247, 263, 328
National Alliance for Nutrition
    and Activity (NANA), 83
National Automatic Merchandising
    Association, 332
National Cancer Institute, 260
National Conference of State Leg-
    islatures, 361
National Dairy Council, 187–88
National Farm to School Program,
    356
National Restaurant Association
    (NRA), xx–xxi, 196–99, 285,
    287, 332, 361
National Soft Drink Association
    (NSDA), 229

natural foods, 26
Nestle, Marion, 52–53, 95–96,
    120, 145, 161, 258
New Mexico, 276
    schools, 235
Newman, Paul, 75
Newman's Own, 75
Nickelodeon, 136–38, 260
nicotine. *See* tobacco industry
No Junk Food program, 358
Nolan, Lucy, 232–33, 343
nonprofit organizations, 62
nutrition-advocacy efforts, xxi, 51
Nutrition Facts law, 203–4
nutrition labeling, 98, 203–4,
    339–42
nutriwashing, 68, 91, 301

O
obesity, 305–9, 342
    childhood, xiv, 307–8, 314
    lawsuits, 275
    surgeon general, 154–56
Obesity Issue Kit, 287
Obesity Working Group, 151
O'Donnell, Daniel, 208–9
Oldways Preservation Trust,
    190–91
Olinto, Jon, 214
Oliver, Jamie, 241, 359
opportunity, 328
Oregon Public Health Institute, 358
Oregon schools, 235–36
Organic Consumers Association,
    357
organizations for change, 355–61
Ornish, Dean, 180
Ortiz, Deborah, 211, 219, 225–27
Ortiz, Felix, 195–96, 205–9, 217
Outback Steakhouse, 64

P

package labeling, 195–217
parents, 27–28, 261–65, 268, 328, 345–46
Parents' Action for Children, 108
Parents Against Junk Food, 356
part of the solution, 328
Passport to Play program, 35, 335
Paull, Matthew, 67, 80–81
Peleo-Lazar, Marlena, 35
People for the Ethical Treatment of Animals (PETA), 54, 59
The People's Grocery, 259
PepsiCo.
  education, 38
  food pyramid, 148
  globalization, 310
  lobbying, 231
  marketing to children, 221, 234
  playgrounds, 33–34
  public relations, 18, 31–33, 180
  Smart Spot program, 99–107, 112
Perdue Farms, 64
Perry, Jim, 128
personal responsibility, xvii, 21–29, 43–44, 161, 288, 306, 328
Personal Responsibility and Work Opportunity Reconciliation Act of 1996, 22
The Personal Responsibility in Food Consumption Act, 288
persuasive intent, 118, 249
Pertschuk, Michael, 252–53
"Pestering Parents: How Food Companies Market Obesity to Children", 247
philanthropy, 32–33
Philip Morris, 46, 62, 107, 124
physical activity, 308

Physician's Committee for Responsible Medicine (PCRM), xxii, 47, 72, 187, 282–83, 357
Pilgrim's Pride, 64
Pizza and Treatza game, 130
playgrounds, 33–34
point of purchase, 328
political frames, xvi
Porter Novelli International, 146
portfolio, 328–29
portion control, 97–98, 197, 329
positives, 329
pouring rights, 123, 221, 325, 346
Poussaint, Alvin F., 77
Powell, Kendall, 94
Powerade, 110
PR Week, 38
preportioning, 97–98
President's Challenge, 336
President's Council on Physical Fitness and Sports, 158–60
press releases, 88–89
presweetened, 329
processed foods, xii–xiii, 91–115
Procter & Gamble, 98
product packaging, 98–100
product placement, 121, 248, 329
profit motive, 4–5
Program on Corporations, Law and Democracy, 361
PRWatch, 63
Public Health Advocacy Institute, 357
public-private partnership, 329
public relations (PR), xiv–xv, 8, 13
Purcell, Amanda, 345

Q

Quaker Oats, 101, 103
Quebec, 266

R

Raines, David, 122
Rajasthan, 189
ReclaimDemocracy.org, 361
reformulation, 329
Reinemund, Steve, 106–7
Rell, Jodi, 230–33
research, 167–94
restaurants, 195–217
    nutrition labeling, 339–42
Riehl, Scott, 286
Rigby, Neville, 267
Right to Eat Enchiladas Act, 276
Ronald McDonald, 34–36
Rosen, Shelly, 21, 31, 154
Rozenich, Anna, 69
Ruby Tuesday, 11, 84
Ruskin, Gary, 183

S

salads, 72–74, 82–85
Salsa, Sabor y Salud, 335
salt, xi, xiii
Sandelman, Bob, 73–74
Satcher, David, 150
Schlosser, Eric, 24
schools
    advertising in, 131–32, 245–71
    resources, 343–49
    soft drinks, 38, 123, 220–44,
        346–49
    See also high schools
Schor, Juliet, 264, 308
Schwarzenegger, Arnold, 228
science, 167–94
self-regulation, 10–13, 329
    advertising, 140–42
Sensible Solutions program, 100,
    108–9, 129, 132–34, 329
Shaping America's Youth, 160, 337

shield laws, 289, 293, 297
Short, Don, 154
silver bullet, 329
Silver, Sheldon, 208
Skinner, Jim, 204
Sloan, Melanie, 62
Small Planet Institute, 357
Smart Brief, 337
S.M.A.R.T. Living, 335
Smart Spot program, 34, 100–6,
    112, 330
Snack Food Association, 332
SnackWell effect, 109
soda. *See* soft drinks
"Soft Drink Hysteria Hard to
    Swallow", 175
soft drinks
    bans in California, 224–26
    consumption, xii–xiii, 170–71
    in schools, 220–44, 346–49
    See also Coca-Cola Company;
        PepsiCo.
"Soft Drinks, Childhood Over-
    weight and the Role of Nutri-
    tion Educators: Let's Base Our
    Solutions on Reality and Sound
    Science", 169–70
sound science, 161, 330
SourceWatch, 63
South Dakota, 276
spin doctoring, 331–37
SpongeBob SquarePants, 131,
    136–39
sports drinks, 109–11, 228
Spurlock, Morgan, 24, 68–69
Stanton, John, 98
stealth marketing, 330
Step With It! curriculum, 39, 335
Stern, Robert, 206–7
Stitt, Kelly, 245

Storey, Maureen, 171
Subway, 72
sugar, xi–xiii, 187
suggestive selling, 330
Sullivan & LeShane, 231
Sullivan, Louis, 180
Sullivan, Patrick, 231
Super Size Me, 24, 68–69, 72, 277
supersizing, 68–69, 72
Supreme Court, 257–58
The Surgeon General's Call to
    Action to Prevent and Decrease
    Overweight and Obesity, 304
Sustain: The Alliance for Better
    Food and Farming, 360
Sweden, 266

T
Taaffe, Ellen, 101–4, 106
target marketing, 75–78
tax-exempt organizations, 62
television
    advertising, 119, 122, 248,
        252–53
    Canada, 266
    Ireland, 266
    Sweden, 266, 268
third-party experts, 330
Thompson, Tommy, xvii–xix, 71,
    143, 150–54, 234, 260
Thorsgaard, Marybeth, 95, 120
Time/ABC Summit on Obesity,
    154
Time magazine, 156
tobacco industry
    bans, 257, 268, 303, 305–6
    globalization, 309
    litigation, 276, 282–83
    tactics, 43, 226
    zoning laws, 270

tort reform, 330
toy bans, 270
trans fat, 12, 70–71, 96–97
trial lawyers, 330
    See also litigation
Tropicana, 101
Tyson Foods, 64

U
U.S. Department of Agriculture
    (USDA), 144

V
value meal marketing, 83
Van Riper, Tom, 80–81
vegan, 53
vegetables, xii, 144
Vending Market Watch, 15
veto vote, 82
Viacom, 260
video games, 129–30, 248–49
    See also advergaming
Vilsack, Tom, 16
viral marketing, 324

W
Wartella, Ellen, 250
Washington, D.C. schools, 236
Washington Legal Foundation,
    333
Washington state schools, 236
Weber Shandwick, 38
Weekly Reader MyPyramid, 336
weight-loss obsession, 306–7
Weight Watchers, 306
Weinberg Group, 168
Weissman, Robert, 185
Wendy's International, 64
Westen, Tracy, 252–53, 255, 258
Whelan, Elizabeth, 178

white flour, 92–93
Whitman, Bill, 79, 81
Whole Foods, 26
whole grains, 92–97, 144
Whole Grains Council, 191, 333
Widmeyer Communications, 39
Wilber, Tricia, 128
Williams, Donald, 233
Williams, Venus, 76–77
Wootan, Margo, 262
World Health Organization, 268
Worldwide Health & Wellness
    Advisory Council, 181, 334
Wyoming, 276

Y
"A Year of Public Health Lunacy",
    178
Yoplait yogurt, 187
Your Power to Choose program,
    237
Yum Brands, 309–10

Z
Zemel, Michael, 187